Marriage and Fertility Behaviour in Japan

Nobutaka Fukuda

Marriage and Fertility Behaviour in Japan

Economic Status and Value-Orientation

Springer

Nobutaka Fukuda
Tohoku University
Sendai
Miyagi
Japan

ISBN 978-981-10-0292-2 ISBN 978-981-10-0294-6 (eBook)
DOI 10.1007/978-981-10-0294-6

Library of Congress Control Number: 2015958326

Printed on acid-free paper

This Springer imprint is published by SpringerNature
The registered company is Springer Science+Business Media Singapore Pte Ltd.

Sirogane mo
Kugane mo tama mo
Nanisemuni
Masareru takara
Ko ni sikame ya mo

(*Man'yō-shū,* V. xi)

My translation
What is the use
Of securing silver
Or gold or sapphire?
What can be more precious
Than a jewel of a child?

Acknowledgements

The roots of this book go back to my doctoral thesis at the University of Oxford, and I wish to express great thanks to all the people who have contributed to its evolution over several years. I would first like to thank my supervisors at Oxford: David Colman, Richard Smith, and Sheila Johansson. Their critical and constructive comments undoubtedly enriched and heightened the scope of this study. My deep gratitude also goes to Ron Lesthaeghe and Osamu Saito for their very insightful comments and suggestions on family formation in Europe and Japan. I am also grateful to good fellows and colleagues: Eva Bernhardt, Jonathan Bradshaw, Ann Gauthier, Jenny Gierveld, Roger Goodman, Andrew Hinde, John Hobcraft, Jan Hoem, Dirk van de Kaa, John Landers, James McMullen, Arthur Stockwin, Ann Waswo, Christopher Wilson, and Anthony Wrigley. They all generously gave me helpful advice and comments on this study.

I started to write this book at Chicago and finished it at Berkeley. I would like to thank Kazuo Yamaguchi (University of Chicago) and John Lie (University of California, Berkeley) for many stimulating conversations concerning this study and for giving me a wonderful research environment. My research stays at Chicago and Berkeley were financially supported by the Abe Fellowship, and the data I used in this study are part of the Japanese Generations and Gender Project. I extend my gratitude to all members of this research project. I am also indebted to Margaret Shade for her editorial help. I would finally like to express thanks to Ryoichi Miwa for his warm support and kindness.

Contents

Author Biography

Nobutaka Fukuda is a professor at Tohoku University, Japan, where he teaches Sociology and Social Statistics. He was a visiting researcher at the University of Oxford in 2000, the University of Chicago in 2012, and the University of California, Berkeley, in 2014. After obtaining his BA in Economics and MA in Sociology of Education in Japan, he continued his research into Japanese Family at the University of Oxford. He received his doctorate from the University of Oxford, and writes many articles and books concerning Japanese family. He is one of the leading researchers on low fertility in Japan, and studies the relation between family formation and ideational change caused by socio-economic development. He is currently working on a comparative study of partnership, fertility, and intergenerational relations between Japan and other developed countries.

Chapter 1
Introduction

1.1 Demographic Developments in Developed Countries

In The Communist Manifesto (1848), Karl Marx and Friedrich Engels stated, "A spectre is haunting Europe—the spectre of Communism". This spectre has now been exorcised in European countries. Nowadays, the economy, despite its lack of a moral ability to cultivate a sense of *noblesse oblige*, is running on a market system in these countries. Instead, another spectre is haunting European and East Asian developed countries—the spectre of anti-natalism and anti-maritalism. After the end of the post-war Baby Boom, a marked decline in fertility has been seen in these countries, albeit with variations in tempo and level, while marriage has been saliently losing its popularity as a form of partnership relation. Indeed, the total period fertility rate (TPFR) in many European countries started to decline in the late 1960s and continues to stay below the replacement level of population size (Coleman 1996; Esping-Andersen and Billari 2015). In the same vein, Japan has been experiencing a drop in its TPFR from the mid 1970s onwards in tandem with a rise in mean age at marriage, whereas Hong Kong, Singapore, South Korea, and Taiwan also reached a below-replacement level of fertility in the 1980s (Frejka et al. 2010; Suzuki 2013). If this trend continues, these countries will, sooner or latter, experience population shrinkage alongside a skewness in age structure.

Admittedly, fears of population decline caused by a scarcity of births have been harboured in the past by European countries such as France (Gauthier 1993; Spengler 1938; Teitelbaum and Winter 1985). However, the current decline in fertility as seen in developed countries differs strikingly from previously experienced periods of decline in its profound and far-reaching impact on our society. In particular, the continuation of the low fertility rate will produce a population with relatively fewer young people and relatively more elderly people in the absence

N. Fukuda, *Marriage and Fertility Behaviour in Japan*,
DOI 10.1007/978-981-10-0294-6_1

of massive immigration. Furthermore, due to progress in medical knowledge and improvements in hygiene and nutrition standards, life expectancy is increasing to an unprecedentedly high level. These changes lead to an increase in unbalanced and ageing populations, which will undoubtedly necessitate the reconstruction of public welfare and social security systems.

Japan is not an exception. The Japanese TPFR fell from 2.13 in 1970 to 1.41 in 2012 with a reduction of 33.8 %, while the mean age at first marriage rose from 26.9 to 30.8 for men and from 24.2 to 29.2 for women during the same period (for details, see Chaps. 3 and 4). It was particularly surprising that the TPFR plunged to 1.57 in 1989, a rate even lower than the 1.58 TPFR experienced in 1966, the Year of the Fire Horse. To elaborate, it is traditionally held in Japan that daughters born in the Year of the Fire Horse bring misfortune, so there is a powerful tendency among the Japanese to avoid giving birth to children in that year (Taeuber 1958; The Population Problems Research Council 1994). Thus, the fact that the TPFR in 1989 was even lower than the 1966 fire-horse-year figure of 1.58 caused increasing social concern about the decline of the fertility rate in Japan. Since the Japanese TPFR reached this astonishingly low level, it has been repeatedly mentioned that fertility decline and ageing population will bring negative impacts on Japanese society such as an economic decline caused by a labour force shortage and a breakdown in the pension system for the elderly (Matsutani 2006). In fact, the percentage of people aged over 65 in Japan's total population reached fully 24.1 % in 2012.

Driven by similar demographic circumstances, many developed countries have implemented a variety of policies in order to increase the number of births and to impede the progress of population ageing (Gauthier 1996; Kaufmann et al. 1997, 2002; Luci-Greulich and Thévenon 2013; McDonald 2006; Moors and Palomba 1995, 1998; Noin and Woods 1993). Indeed, governmental policy intervention includes the fields of social welfare, employment relations, and benefits in cash and kind, ranging from maternity and parental leave to family allowance to childcare services. Japan is not an exceptional case. Its government has been implementing pronatalist policies, comprising the so-called Angel Plan, since the mid-1990s. This package of Japanese governmental measures to encourage people to have children includes an extension of parental leave and an increase in child benefits and childcare provisions, although their pronatal effects have not yet been observed clearly. Hence, it is safe to say that the impact of such policies on patterns of partnership and family formation still remains to be seen (Harknett et al. 2014; Gauthier 2007; Gauthier and Philipo 2008). It is, indeed, unclear whether Sweden's relatively high fertility rate may be attributable to generous public and welfare policies or whether it actually derives from a family–friendly culture in a society that has been sustained by a whole raft of various policies over time (Hoem 2008). Despite such uncertainties, it is crystal clear that marriage and fertility patterns manifest themselves as a social issue in contemporary Japan.

1.2 Social Science and Demographic Behaviour

At the same time, it should not be overlooked that the underlying causes of changes in marriage and fertility behaviour have been hitherto clarified insufficiently in Japan. At a superficial glance, we can easily find a good description of these changes from the viewpoint of formal demography. To be specific, this descriptive approach, utilizing mechanical decomposition, holds that the level of fertility is composed of nine proximate determinants such as the percentage of married women and the use of contraception (Bongaarts and Potter 1983). According to adherents of this approach, a fluctuation in the level of fertility is related solely to a change in these proximate determinants. For instance, the TPFR is broken down by this method into the marriage rate, the marital fertility rate, and the extramarital birth rate (Gupta 1993). Accordingly, a decline in the TPFR is almost completely attributed to shrinkage in the proportion of married adults as long as intra- and extra-marital births remain unchanged. This decomposition approach is often utilized to provide an exposition of Japanese fertility decline. For example, as will be shown in the following chapters, Japan has an extremely small number of extramarital births. Those adhering to this decomposition approach tenaciously insist that the fall in the Japanese TPFR has been caused almost singlehandedly by a decrease in the marriage rate. Along the same lines, adherents to this approach maintain that the dissemination of effective contraceptive methods was, in effect, entirely responsible for the small size of families in the USA (Westoff and Ryder 1977). This method was also applied in the analysis of the change in marriage patterns. Their conclusions in this instance put forward, for example, that a decline in nuptiality may be attributable to an imbalanced sex ratio between men and women at marriageable age (Guttentag and Secord 1983).

Admittedly, the results of a decomposition approach show, in a simple and straightforward way, a covariant relation between marriage and fertility, contraception and fertility, and sex ratio and marriage (Morgan and Tayor 2006). In fact, breaking down the TPFR into its nuptiality and marital-birth constituents can bring us closer to an intuitive understanding of fertility change. Such arithmetic techniques, however, provide us with nothing more than elaborate descriptions (Hobcraft 2002). They neither explain the socio-economic reasons for demographic changes nor show a causal relation between social factors and human behaviour at all (McNicoll 1992). In this sense, the decomposition approach is confined to formal and mechanical illustrations of marriage and fertility patterns. This approach ultimately leaves us far from a social scientific understanding of human behaviour.

What we should not forget here is that human behaviours are not performed within a societal vacuum. More specifically, whatever action may be taken in a society, it is related to social conditions and contexts. It therefore follows that an individual action in a human society is well understood only when its mechanisms are analysed and explicated by social factors. Hence, the societal forces behind human conduct need to be clarified as much as possible from a social sciences standpoint. Émile Durkheim's analysis of suicide is a case in point. While suicide is in itself an individual action, its causes cannot be totalized or made entirely attributable to personal factors. Rather, the mechanisms underlying the incidence of suicide as an aspect of human conduct need to be understood and explicated as a societal phenomenon through the application of the interpretive tools and methods of the social sciences (Durkheim 1982, 2006). Otherwise, an individual action will be analysed in the same way that physical science deals with, resulting in a purely asocial explanation of human conduct that provides a meagre contribution at best towards increasing our understanding. In sum, from a social sciences viewpoint, it is necessary to clarify the social factors that drive people to take specific actions and to understand the social structures that circumscribe the range of people's behavioural choices.

The same holds true for studies on marriage and fertility behaviour. Admittedly, biological and technological elements, as exemplified by demographic decomposition methods, affect feasibility and variability in the behavioural choice of marriage and childbearing. It is likely that these factors are associated with one's decisions on partnership and family formation. At the same time, however, the feasibility and variability of human conduct is constructed, recognized, and evaluated by people within a society. We can therefore argue that there are no biological, technological, and compositional influences beyond one's choice of action. In this sense, whatever choice is made, the decision depends ultimately on the social conditions and contexts in which people live. Hence, as long as we limit ourselves to the decomposition approach, it will be almost impossible to arrive at social scientific explications for marriage and fertility patterns. Taking these points into consideration, one can see that, in order to arrive at a clear understanding of social scientific causation, it is necessary to link our societal factors to demographic behaviour, based on social theories of human behaviour. As Ansley Coale put it, a specific form of demographic behaviour is neither adopted nor disseminated until societal circumstances generate the readiness and willingness for it (Coale 1973; Lesthaeghe and Vanderhoeft 2001).

1.3 Marriage and Childbearing Patterns in Japan

When it comes down to a theoretical framework, two basic factors—economic and ideational—are noteworthy when explicating marriage and fertility behaviour in developed countries (Morgan and Taylor 2006), and it is safe to say that economic and ideational changes play a key role in determining the patterns of partnership and family formation in these countries. As will be discussed in Chap. 2, these theoretical frameworks may be regarded as putative and appropriate from a viewpoint of social action theory. Furthermore, the impact of these two factors on marriage and fertility behaviour has commanded much scholarly interest to date and provided subject matter for a great deal of empirical research. More specifically, while particular attention has been given to the causal relation between the direct and the opportunity costs of having children, the influence of young adults' earning capability has also been investigated in research on marriage patterns from an economic point of view. In the same vein, as far as ideational changes are concerned, a value shift has been seen as an underlying cause in recent changes pertaining to partnership and family formation in European countries after the late 1960s (for details, see Chap. 2).

Turning to prior studies on marriage and fertilityFertility patterns in Japan, the influence of economic change has attracted much scholarly attention. As is well known, Japan experienced unprecedented economic growth in the post-war period, which undoubtedly led to the extraordinary transformation of its socio-economic structures. In particular, the extent of this transformation can be easily recognized in the shift of women's socio-economic status (Brinton 1993). Undoubtedly, an increase in educational levels and employment opportunities should have served to better women's economic empowerment in the public sphere. Kindled by such a post-war social situation, research interest has hitherto become focused mainly on the impact of economic factors on Japanese marriage and fertility patterns. For example, the influence of male and female wages on the level of fertility has been the subject of much investigation in the post-war period in Japan (Hashimoto 1974, 1980; Ohbuchi 1982; Ogawa and Mason 1986; Ogawa et al. 2009; Osawa 1988). Likewise, a great deal of research has been expended on the relation between women's earning capability and marriage (Ermisch and Ogawa 1994; Retherford et al. 2001; Zuanna et al. 1998). Moreover, academic interest along the same line has motivated researchers to carry out investigations concerning the impact of economic factors on marriage and childbearing patterns in pre-war Japan (Mosk 1980, 1983).

By contrast, sufficient examination has not been carried out regarding the impact of ideational factors on marriage and fertility patterns in Japan. While it is maintained that a value shift has no influence on Japanese marriage and childbearing patterns (Retherford et al. 1996; Retherford and Ogawa 2006), most of these claims are based on superficial descriptions of survey data and not on the sharp and sufficiently detailed analysis of demographic patterns. Hence, it is premature to conclude that attitudinal factors have no influence on marriage and fertility behaviour in Japan. Besides, it is also pointed out that ideational and attitudinal factors affect the patterns of Japanese partnership and family formation (Atoh 2008a, b; Hodge and Ogawa 1991). In fact, many survey results show that attitudes towards gender, partnership, and family relations have been changing in Japan (Choe et al. 2014; Rindfuss et al. 2004; Tsuya and Bumpass 2004; Tsuya and Mason 1995). This evidence suggests that a value shift has a bearing on marriage and fertility behaviour in contemporary Japan. Furthermore, as we will discuss in detail in the following chapters, it is very likely that economic development has caused, and is continuing to cause, ideational, and attitudinal changes in developed countries such as Japan. Hence, we can argue that sufficient light will never be shed on the mechanisms of partnership and family formation in contemporary Japan as long as we continue to look only at the influence of economic factors. Rather, a dynamic analysis of economic and ideational factors is essential in order to fully understand the social determinants of Japanese marriage and fertility behaviour.

In addition, it should be borne in mind that the theoretical framework of marriage and fertility owes its origins to Western society. Indeed, economic theories of marriage and fertility were developed mainly in the USA, while the impact of a value shift on partnership and family formation was first proposed in the Netherlands and Belgium (for details, see Chap. 2). The development of these analytical frameworks is undoubtedly affected by the historical experiences and cultural contexts of these specific countries. Hence, it may very well be that these theories do not possess the appropriate social, cultural, or historical framework required to shed any fresh light on marriage and childbearing patterns in Japan. Indeed, it has been pointed out that human conduct and corporate behaviour is constrained by the existing conditions and institutional contexts of a given society (Garrouste and Ioannides 2001). Further, there is no guarantee that non-Western countries follow the same course of demographic development as Western countries (Thornton 2005). Hence, it is necessary to assess the validity of theories concerning Japanese marriage and fertility behaviour carefully.

Taking the discussion thus far into consideration, we can state the two main themes of this book. In concrete terms, the first purpose of this book is to examine the influence of economic and ideational factors on Japanese marriage and fertility behaviour according to the theory of social action. As has already been mentioned, economic and ideational frameworks can be regarded as the most appropriate tools for the social scientific analysis of marriage and childbearing patterns. At the same time, however, these approaches can be highly nuanced by the historical experiences and social contexts of their origins. Thus, entailed in the first purpose of this book are the examination and evaluation of the relevance of these frameworks to the study of Japanese marriage and fertility behaviour. The second purpose of this volume is to investigate a historical transformation in attitudes towards partnership and family in Japan. While scholarly research on Japanese demographic patterns tends to slant towards the influence of economic changes, attitudinal change has hardly been examined at all, particularly from a long historical perspective. This lacuna holds at present despite the fact that the patterns of partnership and family formation have experienced a marked transformation in Japan over the last few decades. Hence, it is essential that we investigate these historical changes in values and attitudes sufficiently and satisfactorily. Particularly in the light of the fact that it has received little attention to date, our examination of a value shift in Japan becomes an imperative.

1.4 Organization of the Book

Having presented the various matters related to this study, it will be useful to outline briefly the structure of this book. Chapter 2 will review recent theories of marriage and fertility behaviour and propose a theoretical framework for use in this study. In particular, the discussion will focus on clarifying the similarities and dissimilarities of the economic and ideational theories of demographic behaviour from a viewpoint of social action theory. Chapter 3 will investigate marriage behaviour in Japan. As mentioned earlier, since Japanese marriage patterns have transformed in tandem with its fertility patterns, this chapter will examine the extent to which economic and attitudinal factors have affected recent marriage behaviour by using the longitudinal data of panel surveys. Chapter 4 will be devoted to the examination of Japanese fertility patterns. More specifically, the chapter will investigate the influence of economic and attitudinal factors on fertility behaviour. The main purpose of Chap. 5 will be the examination of a change in attitudes towards partnership and family relations in Japan by using data from repeated cross-sectional surveys. By analysing a value shift from the aspects of age, cohorts, and periods, Chap. 5 will, in detail, consider both stability and change in attitudes towards partnership and family relations in Japan. In Chap. 6, we will bring together the major findings of the preceding chapters and present our conclusions about the determinants of recent Japanese marriage and fertility behaviour.

References

Atoh, M. (2008a). Family changes in the context of lowest-low fertility: The case of Japan. *International Journal of Japanese Sociology, 17*, 14–29.

Atoh, M. (2008b). The relevance of ideational changes to family transformation in postwar Japan. In R. Jayakody, R. Thornton & W. Axinn (Eds.), *International family change: Ideational perspectives* (pp. 223–250). New York: Lawrence Erlbaum Associates.

Bongaarts, J., & Potter, R. G. (1983). *Fertility, biology and behavior: An analysis of the proximate determinants*. New York: Academic Press.

Brinton, M. C. (1993). *Women and the economic miracle: Gender and work in the postwar Japan*. Berkeley: University of California Press.

Choe, M. K., Bumpass, L. L., Tsuya, N. O., & Rindfuss, R. R. (2014). Nontraditional family-related attitudes in Japan: Macro and micro determinants. *Population and Development Review, 40*, 241–271.

Coale, A. J. (1973). The demographic transition reconsidered. In *Proceedings of the International Population Conference, Liège, 1973* (pp.53–72). Liège: International Union for the Scientific Study of Population.

Coleman, D. (Ed.). (1996). *Europe's population in the 1990s*. Oxford: Oxford University Press.

Gupta, P. D. (1993). *Standardization and decomposition of rates*. Washington, DC: US Government Printing Office.

Durkheim, É. (1982). *The rules of sociological method*. New York: Free Press.

Durkheim, É. (2006). *On suicide*. New York: Penguin Books.

Ermisch, J., & Ogawa, N. (1994). Age at motherhood in Japan. *Journal of Population Economics, 7*, 393–420.

Esping-Andersen, G., & Billari, F. C. (2015). Re-theorizing family demographics. *Population and Development Review, 41*(1), 1–31.

Frejka, T., Jones, G. W., & Sardon, J. P. (2010). East Asian childbearing patterns and policy developments. *Population and Development Review, 36*, 579–606.

Garrouste, P., & Ioannides, S. (Eds.). (2001). *Evolution and path dependence in economic ideas: Past and present*. Cheltenham: Edward Elgar.

Gauthier, A. H. (1993). Towards renewed fears of population and family decline. *European Journal of Population, 9*, 143–168.

Gauthier, A. H. (1996). *The state and the family*. Oxford: Clarendon Press.

Gauthier, A. H. (2007). The impact of family policies on fertility in industrialized countries: A review of the literature. *Population Research and Policy Review, 26*, 323–346.

Gauthier, A. H., & Philipov, D. (2008). Can policies enhance fertility in Europe? *Vienna Yearbook of Population Research, 2008*, 1–16.

Guttentag, M., & Secord, P. F. (1983). *Too many women?: The sex ratio question*. Newbury Park: SAGE Publications.

Harknett, K., Billari, F. C., & Medalia, C. (2014). Do family support environments influence fertility? *European Journal of Population, 30*, 1–33.

Hashimoto, M. (1974). Economics of postwar fertility in Japan. *Journal of Political Economy, 82*, S170–S194.

Hashimoto, M. (1980). Demand for children in Japan during modernization. *Research in Population Economics, 2*, 295–320.

Hobcraft, J. (2002). Moving beyond elaborate description: Towards understanding choices about parenthood. In M. Macura & G. Beets (Eds.), *Dynamics of fertility and partnership in Europe: Insights and lessons from comparative research* (pp. 131–143). New York: United Nations.

Hodge, R. W., & Ogawa, N. (1991). *Fertility change in contemporary Japan*. Chicago: University of Chicago Press.

Hoem, J. M. (2008). The impact of public policies on European fertility. *Demographic Research, 19*(10), 249–260.

Kaufmann, F. X., Kuijsten, A., Sheulze, H. J., & Strohmeier, K. P. (Eds.). (1997). *Family life and family policies in Europe volume 1: Structures and trends in the 1980s*. Oxford: Clarendon Press.

Kaufmann, F. X., Kuijsten, A., Sheulze, H. J., & Strohmeier, K. P. (Eds.). (2002). *Family life and family policies in Europe volume 2: Problems and issues in comparative perspective*. Oxford: Oxford University Press.

Lesthaeghe, R., & Vanderhoeft, C. (2001). Ready, willing, and able: A conceptualization of transitions to new behavioral forms. In J. B. Casterline (Eds.), *Diffusion processes and fertility transition* (pp. 240–264). Washington D.C.: National Academy Press.

Luci-Greulich, A., & Thévenon, O. (2013). The impact of family policies on fertility trends in developed countries. *European Journal of Population, 29*(4), 387–416.

Matsutani, A. (2006). *Shrinking-population economics: Lessons from Japan*. Tokyo: International House of Japan.

McDonald, P. (2006). An assessment of policies that support having children from the perspectives of equity, efficiency and efficacy. *Vienna Yearbook of Population Research, 2006*, 213–234.

McNicoll, G. (1992). The agenda of population studies: A commentary and complaint. *Population and Development Review, 18*, 399–420.

Moors, H., & Palomba, R. (Eds.). (1995). *Population, family, and welfare: A comparative survey of European attitudes* (Vol. 1). Oxford: Clarendon Press.

Moors, H., & Palomba, R. (Eds.). (1998). *Population, family, and welfare: A comparative survey of European attitudes* (Vol. 2). Oxford: Clarendon Press.

Morgan, S. P. & Taylor, M. G. (2006). Low Fertility at the Turn of the Twenty-First Century. *Annual Review of Sociology, 32*, 375–399.

Mosk, C. (1980). Nuptiality in Meiji Japan. *Journal of Social History, 13*, 474–489.

Mosk, C. (1983). *Patriarchy and fertility: Japan and Sweden, 1880–1960*. New York: Academic Press.

Noin, D., & Woods, R. (Eds.). (1993). *The changing of population of Europe*. Oxford: Blackwell.

Ogawa, N., & Mason, A. (1986). An economic analysis of recent fertility in Japan: An application of the Butz-Ward model. *Journal of Population Studies, 9*, 5–14.

Ogawa, N., Retherford, R. D., & Matsukura, R. (2009). Japan's declining fertility and policy responses. In G. Jones, P. T. Straughan & A. Chan (Eds.), *Ultra-low fertility in Pacific Asia: Trends, causes and policy issues* (pp. 40–72). London: Routledge.

Ohbuchi, H. (1982). Empirical tests of the chicago model and the easterline hypothesis: A case study of Japan. *Journal of Population Studies, 5*, 8–16.

Osawa, M. (1988). Working mothers: Changing patterns of employment and fertility in Japan. *Economic Development and Cultural Change, 36*, 623–650.

Retherford, R., & Ogawa, N. (2006). Japan's baby bust: Cause, implications, and policy responses. In F. R. Harris (Eds.), *The baby bust: Who will do the work? Who will pay the taxes?* (pp. 5–47). Lanham, Maryland: Rowman & Littlefielf Publishers.

Retherford, R., Ogawa, N., & Sakamoto, S. (1996). Values and fertility change in Japan. *Population Studies, 50*, 5–25.

Retherford, R. D., Ogawa, N., & Matsukura, R. (2001). Late marriage and less marriage in Japan. *Population and Development Review, 27*, 65–102.

Rindfuss, R. R., Choe, M. K., Bumpass, L. L., & Tsuya, N. O. (2004). Social networks and family change in Japan. *American Sociological Review, 69*, 838–861.

Spengler, J. J. (1938). *France faces depopulation*. Durham: Duke University Press.

Suzuki, T. (2013). *Low fertility and population Aging in Japan and East Asia*. Tokyo: Springer.

Taeuber, I. B. (1958). *The population of Japan*. Princeton: Princeton University Press.

Teitelbaum, M. S., & Winter, Jay M. (1985). *The fear of population decline*. Orland: Academic Press.

The Population Problems Research Council, (Ed.). (1994). *The population and society of post-war Japan*. Tokyo: Mainichi Newspapers.

Thornton, A. (2005). *Reading history sideways: The fallacy and enduring impact on the developmental paradigm on family life*. Chicago: The University of Chicago Press.

Tsuya, N. O., & Bumpass, L. L. (Eds.). (2004). *Marriage, work, and family life in comparative perspective: Japan, South Korea, and the United States*. Honolulu: University of Hawaii Press.

Tsuya, N. O., & Mason, K. O. (1995). Changing gender roles and below-replacement fertility in Japan. In K. O. Mason & A. M. Jensen (Eds.), *Gender and family change in industrialized countries* (pp. 139–167). Oxford: Clarendon Press.

Westoff, C. F., & Ryder, N. B. (1977). *Contraceptive revolution*. Princeton: Princeton University Press.

Zuanna, G. D., Atho, M., Castiglioni, M., & Kojima, K. (1998). Late marriage among young people: The case of Italy and Japan. *Genus, LIV*, 187–232.

Chapter 2
Economic and Ideational Theories of Marriage and Fertility Behaviour

2.1 Introduction

The purpose of this chapter is to reconsider marriage and fertility behaviour in developed countries from a viewpoint of social action theory. A number of decades ago, Duesenbery (1960) stated, "Economics is all about how people make choices. Sociology is all about why they don't have any choices to make". This remark aptly describes a difference in the analytical framework of fertility fertility behaviour between the two academic disciplines. On the one hand, an economist sees demographic behaviour as the process of arranging material conditions to maximize one's utility (satisfaction). On the other hand, a sociologist focuses on values and norms that encourage or discourage people to take a specific action. The former's scholarly concern lies in optimizing instrumental resources to attain a fixed goal (preference); the latter is interested in the beliefs and regulations that provide the orientation of an individual action.

A similar contrast is seen in interpretations of demographic phenomena after the late 1960s. As is well known, developed countries experienced a marked change in their patterns of partnership and fertility following the "baby boom" years, which ran from the early 1950s through the early 1960s. After the end of baby boom, the number of cohabiting couples increased substantially in these countries while marriage fell out of favour. During this same period, the level of fertility declined while the the timing of childbirth was postponed. These changes from the second half of the 1960s onwards are often generically termed the "Second Demographic Transition (SDT)" (Lesthaeghe 1983, 1995; van de Kaa 1987, 1994), although a unanimous consensus has not necessary been built on its conceptual appropriateness (Bernhardt 2004; Caldwell 2006). For instance, Cliquet (1991) rejecting the notion of a "Second Demographic Transition", contends that demographic changes after the baby boom can be regarded as part of a process that has been going on over the past several decades. In a similar vein, Coleman (2004)

N. Fukuda, *Marriage and Fertility Behaviour in Japan*,
DOI 10.1007/978-981-10-0294-6_2

claims that these recent demographic phenomena do not fall into the category of a demographic transition and may be more accurately regarded as a preference transition in lifestyle.

Putting aside the conceptual validity of the SDT, no one denies that entering a married status and bearing children are human actions conducted within a society. Thus, the patterns of marriage and fertility in developed countries need to be accounted for fundamentally from a viewpoint of social action (Morgan and Taylor 2006), although some interpretations by mechanical and formal demography have been proposed so far. Taking this point into account, foremost attention should be paid to two contrasting theoretical paths, namely, the economic and ideational theories. Generally speaking, the economic theory holds that, given a fixed preference, objective and material resources such as incomes and employment opportunities determine the demographic patterns and trends of developed countries (McNicoll 1992). The ideational theory, in contrast, places more importance on subjective factors such as human ideas and attitudes towards family and lifestyle than on material conditions as the determinants of demographic behaviour.

It can be easily recognized that these two theories fundamentally differ in their models of human behaviour. More specifically, economic theory assumes that, since human beings are of a materialistic nature, their behaviour hinges on their physical situation. By contrast, ideational theory holds that human beings are oriented towards their values and beliefs, which motivate their actions in specific directions. One must bear in mind, however, that every academic discipline in the social sciences espouses its own model of human behaviour. Admittedly, the framework of a model in the social sciences can eliminate peripheral and residual elements and provide useful guidance for the analysis and better understanding of human behaviour and conduct. Thus, a behavioural model is a useful tool in the interpretation of complex phenomena as long as it is constructed not to replicate human nature, but to utilize as an abstract entity (Simion 1985). At the same time, however, the model must contribute towards getting a precise grasp on reality, and a human subject assumed by the model should be no imaginary creature, but an actual human being, tangibly connected to the complexities of the real world. In other words, the model of human action needs to reflect the way people actually behave in daily life (de Bruijn 1999). These features of a behavioural model necessitate the raising of questions concerning the methodology and epistemology behind the model itself. The model must reflect human behaviour and conduct in the real world in a down-to-earth and recognizable manner. At the same time, however, the model needs be constructed succinctly to delineate the complexities of reality as simply, clearly, and accurately as possible. Thus, a balance between what is real and what is abstract is important for constructing a theoretical model of human behaviour. Moreover, the theoretical model should be evaluated on its relevance to reality and be elaborated upon to enhance its explanatory power.

As already mentioned, economic and ideational theories hold contrasting models of human behaviour in the investigation of marriage and fertility patterns. We should, however, not forget that both disciplines deal with the same research objects. Although the models of these two theories stand at a distinct remove from each other, their conceptual framework of human action is created from the identical social phenomena. Hence, this distance is undoubtedly derived from the fact that the models are constructed in contrasting methods of abstracting reality. At the same time, however, it should also be recognized here that the juxtaposition of many differing theoretical models does not serve in obtaining a clear understanding of the mechanism of marriage and fertility. Rather, since behavioural models are meant to be used as tools for grasping the social phenomena of our world, they should be reconstructed in such a way as to give us a more insightful and inclusive understanding of social reality.

Taking these points into consideration, in this chapter, we will attempt to reconsider a theory of marriage and fertility behaviour from a viewpoint of social action theory. In the following part of the chapter, we will first provide a review on the theory of the SDT. Next, we will move on to discuss the differences between ideational and economic approaches to the explanation of marriage and fertility behaviour. Subsequently, the two behavioural models will be discussed from a viewpoint of rational choice theory, followed by a discussion of the influence of institutional contexts on marriage and fertility behaviour. The concluding emphasis of this chapter will be placed on the importance of empirical studies of the two theories.

2.2 Phenomenological Aspects of the Second Demographic Transition

In order to characterize demographic changes in Western Europe after the baby boom, the concept of the SDT was proposed for the first time by Dirk van de Kaa and Ron Lesthaeghe in a Dutch sociology journal in 1986 (van de Kaa 1996, 2003; Lesthaeghe 2010, 2014). This was, however, not the first attempt to formulate a demographic change from a long historical perspective (Kreager 2015). Similar theories had been put forward before its conceptualization. In fact, the term, "demographic transition", which may sometimes be called "the first demographic transition" (FDT), had already been used by Davis (1945) and Notestein (1953), while Thompson (1929) also characterized the relation between a decline in fertility and mortality in a similar fashion.

Nevertheless, the SDT differs in concept from the first transition on two points. Firstly, the FDT is a framework describing a process of moving from one state of equilibrium to another. The theory assumes that a high level of fertility was formerly balanced with that of mortality. However, due to the modernization of a society, once the death rate starts to reduce, the fertility rate also declines in response to the falling mortality rate. As a result, a demographic state of high fertility and mortality shifts to one of low fertility and mortality. In short, the classical theory of the demographic transition indicates a change of demographic regimes in a homeostatic situation, in which population size stays in equilibrium with almost the same number of births and deaths (Wilson 2013).

In contrast, the SDT does not necessarily assume stability in a demographic regime (van de Kaa 1987, 1994; Lesthaeghe 1995, 2001; Lesthaeghe and Willems 1999). In this theory, no assumption is made that a human population always stabilizes with the replacement level of fertility and low mortality after transiting from high fertility and high mortality. As for below-replacement fertility, which may lead to continuous population decline, this is understood in the framework of the SDT to be a hallmark of the demographic regime of present-day affluent societies (McNicoll 2012). Indeed, the total period fertility rate (TPFR) had plunged to the below-replacement level in Europe by the 1980s (Coleman 1996). As it is assumed in the orthodox demographic transition that the number of births and deaths would sooner or later reach equilibrium, the emergent of below-replacement fertility which does not bring that equilibrium was seen as an unexpected and surprising demographic phenomenon (Demeny 1997). This novel situation attracted research interest and much ink has been spilt in describing the features of fertility patterns. For example, "lowest-low fertility" was coined to describe the extreme scarcity of newborn babies in Mediterranean countries (Kohler et al. 2002). In addition, it was pointed out that the postponement of childbirth and recuperation of fertility are the salient features of European reproductive patterns, although there is very little agreement how far recuperation effects will increase the level of fertility (Billari et al. 2006; Lesthaeghe and Permanyer 2014; Lesthaeghe and Willems 1999).

Secondly and more importantly, the SDT includes more far-reaching changes than the first transition in patterns of partnership and family formation after the 1960s. Indeed, patterns of partnership have, albeit with regional variations in speed and extent, changed in tandem with changes in reproductive patterns in European countries. For instance, the number of births out of wedlock has risen in Western and Northern Europe (Kiernan 1996, 1999b). The percentage of extra-marital births over all live births, which stood at less than 10 % in 1970, reached around 50 % in Denmark, France, Norway, the Netherlands and the United Kingdom in 2011, whereas the crude divorce rate, which is affected by the proportion of aged and children's populations, has risen from approximately 1.0 per thousand to 2.0 per thousand in the same period (Eurostat Database). Likewise, cohabitation has also been gaining in popularity as either an alternative or a prelude to marriage in North-western Europe (Kiernan 1999a, 2001, 2004; Ní Bhrolcháin and Beaujouan 2013). Similarly, Latain American countries such as Argentina, Brazil and Chile have also increased the number of cohabitated couples since the 1990s (Esteve et al. 2012). Furthermore, the timing of leaving a natal home has been delayed, reaching nearly age 30 in Southern Europe (Iacovou and Parisi 2009).

These phenomena naturally allow us to move out from the narrow world of the mortality–fertility relationship in Demography. In short, the central focus of the FDT is a shift from one state of equilibrium between mortality and fertility to another state. Even if marriage behaviour is analysed in the FDT, the primary interest lies in its influence on marital fertility. This is because most births occurred within wedlock and nuptiality was tightly linked to fertility. Hence, the FDT does not explicitly deal with transformations in partnership, such as cohabitation and divorce. In this regard, it seems better to view the SDT as not purely demographic but inclusive of changes of partnership and family formation (Coleman 2004). Indeed, van de Kaa (2003) puts forward to a list of fifteen sequential stages observed through the process of the SDT. This list includes changes in reproductive patterns such as sub-replacement fertility, delayed childbearing and premarital birth. At the same time, however, partnership changes seen in phenomena such as the rising divorce rate and the increasing prevalence of cohabitation and the postponement of marriage are referred to as features of the SDT.

These sequential indicators were proposed in order to clarify and universalize the theory of the SDT. With the benefit of hindsight, however, it cannot be denied that they have made the concept of the SDT elusive and ambiguous. For simplicity, let us consider the following cases. Country A displays the last five features in the van de Kaa list without showing evidence of the first five changes, while Country B exhibits only five demographic phenomena from the middle of this same list. In these cases, it is very difficult to judge whether the two countries are undergoing the SDT. In other words, as the descriptive definition of the SDT becomes more strict and rigid, exceptional and irregular cases become more intractable to consider. In fact, looking at only European countries, the case is more complicated than the theory of the SDT expected. For instance, the total period fertility rate (TPFR) shows a salient diverse trend in European countries. Due to the fact that a decline in the TPFR started in the mid-1970s and spread over Europe until the end of the 1990s, a TPFR of below 1.5 (so-called "very low fertility") was observed in 25 out of 39 European countries in 2002. Furthermore, the TPFR of 16 countries stood below 1.3, the so-called lowest-low fertility, among 39 European countries with populations of more than 100,000 in the same year (Kohler et al. 2002). These countries have, however, displayed a diverse trajectory of fertility patterns since the first decade of the twenty-first century (Frejka and Sobotka 2008; Neyer 2013; Sobotka 2008a, b). Western and Northern European countries (excluding German-speaking countries) have the highest low fertility whose TPFR is equal to or more than 1.85. Indeed, the TPFR bounced back to over 1.8 in Belgium, Denmark, Finland, Sweden and the UK in 2011, while it reached even 2.0 in France. In contrast, Eastern European countries such as Hungary and Poland, and Southern European countries such as Italy and Spain still remained at a very low fertility, with TPFRs staying around 1.5 in 2011. Furthermore, the TPFR level fluctuated at around 1.3 among East Asian developed countries such as Japan, South Korea, Singapore and Taiwan (Goldstein et al. 2009). These regional variations on fertility patterns sketch scenarios other than those expected by the SDT. The same holds true in patterns of living arrangements and partnership formation. An increase in the number of cohabitations and extra-marital births is regarded as one of the important signals which indicate that a country has entered the stage of the SDT. Developed countries, however, show regional variations on these demographic indicators. For example, although Romania and the Russian Federation reached a very low fertility, cohabitation did not gain as much in popularity in these two countries as in North-western Europe (Potârca et al. 2013). In particular,

Romanians, like Italians, tend to prefer the postponement or abandonment of legal marriage to cohabitation even in their young birth cohorts. Moreover, the number of extra-marital births has increased in Australia (Carmichael 2014), although the number still remains extremely small in Japan (for details, see Chaps. 3 and 4). Partnership formation and parenthood pattern tend to change simultaneously in Western and Northern Europe, whereas the salient postponement of marriage and childbearing and a mild increase in cohabitation, as a whole, occur in East Asian with a patriarchal family system and Southern Europe. In contrast, Latin American countries show a drastic rise in the number of cohabitations and a modest delay in the timing of childbearing (Esteve et al. 2012; Lesthaeghe 2014).

Apart form the detailed description of geographical variations in partnership and childbearing patterns, it is certain that not only fertility but also marriage patterns differ considerably between developed countries. Undoubtedly, this regional variation calls the universality and pervasiveness of the SDT into question. More specifically, the notion of the SDT has been used to attempt to describe universal features of demographic changes in developed countries after the 1960s, but yet this grand narrative has not yet been developed and elaborated upon to the point where it can be granted universal consent. In short, the patterns of partnership, living arrangements and family building show, for the time being, a great geographical diversity. Hence, we can argue that, on the descriptive side, the theory of the SDT is not so sophisticated as to grasp demographic reality in developed countries accurately and sufficiently.

2.3 Economic Theories of Marriage and Fertility Behaviour

As discussed in the proceeding section, the theory of the SDT lacks sufficient breadth of scope and content to be employed as a general description of demographic phenomena in developed countries after the 1960s. As exemplified by an increase in the number of consensual unions, postponed marriages and extra-marital births, partnership and childbearing patterns have shown more diverse developments in these countries than anticipated in the theory. This evidence naturally challenges the validity of the concept as a comprehensive description of demographic change in industrialized society. At the same time, it should not be, however, overlooked that the theory of the SDT also includes an explanatory framework for demographic behaviour in developed countries. More specifically, this concept aims to put forward a theoretical alternative to Richard Easterlin's and Gery Becker's economic theories regarding marriage and fertility (Lesthaeghe 2010). We will provide a detailed discussion on this point, but before moving on to that, it would be helpful to take a brief look at the economic theories on marriage and fertility behaviour. Since a considerable number of studies on marriage and childbearing behaviour from an economic point of view have been carried out hitherto, it is outside the scope of this chapter to give an exhaustive review of previous research on the economic theory of marriage and family. Rather, in the following discussion, we will concentrate on the theoretical features of economic analysis on marriage and fertility.

Received wisdom has it that the economic theory of marriage and fertility is classified into two groups: New Home Economics theory and Easterlin's theory. The New Home Economics theory on fertility behaviour was initially articulated by Becker (1960) and has been developed mainly by his colleagues (Becker 1976, 1986, 1991, 1996; Becker and Barro 1988; Becker and Lewis 1973; Butz and Ward 1979; Folbre 1996; Rosenzweig and Stark 1997; Schultz 1974; Werding 2014; Willis 1973). Although this theory has been formulated by several authors in various terms, the heart of its theoretical framework lies in its application of the Hicks–Allen consumption theory to fertility behaviour (Androka 1978). Thus, this theory presumes that human fertility behaviour can be equated to human behaviour in the consumption of market goods and services. More specifically, the New Home Economics theory is formulated on the basis of two assumptions. The first assumption is that, in an industrialized society, children are no longer of any productive or economic utility to their parents and can be regarded purely as consumption goods bringing psychological satisfaction to their parents. As Leibenstein (1974, 1975, 1976, 1981) points out, children may have several sorts of utility at a less developed stage of society. For instance, after entering the labour force, children may provide help either on the family's farm or workshop or earn an income to add to the common household fund. In addition, grown-up children may provide subsistence for their aged parents. However, these two forms of utility rarely exist in highly developed society (Caldwell 1982). The theory's second basic assumption holds that a household (or a couple) spends its time and money and consumes goods and services, in order to maximize its utility (satisfaction) in a fixed and stable preference. As mentioned by orthodox modernization theories, one of the most distinctive features of social development from an agrarian to an industrialized society is the functional differentiation of family and household (Burgess and Lock 1945; Ogburn and Nimkoff 1955). In concrete terms, although the family was a unit with many social functions such as protection, education, production and consumption in an agrarian society, it performs very few functions such as children's socialization and the stabilization of adults' personality in an industrialized society (Levy 1966; Moore 1974; Parsons and Bales 1955; Smelser 1959). In view of that, the activities of contemporary families and households are, to a considerable degree, directed towards gaining satisfaction from consuming goods and services. In this sense, the degree to which goods and services bring satisfaction when they are consumed plays an important role in a couple's (or a household's) behaviour.

Based on these assumptions, the New Home Economics theory holds that, under the constraint of its monetary budget, a couple consumes goods in such a way as to maximize their utility in a fixed preference ordering.[1] More concretely,

[1]Becker (1996) attempts to propose a utility function which allows preference to be more dynamic and changeable. Yet, the formation of human preference is, in reality, more complicated than Becker formalizes (for details, see Henrich et al. 2004).

the theory assumes that a rise in household income will, *ceteris paribus*, increase the number of children. This relation easily finds its analogy in the consumption theory in which the level of household income determines the consumption level of market goods and services. At the same time, however, the theory recognizes that a higher income does not always lead to an increase in the demand for children. This may occur when the "substitute effect" outweighs the "income effect". In concrete terms, Becker and and Lewis (1973) formulate this phenomenon as the interaction between the quantity and quality of children. In consumption behaviour, it is likely that, instead of increasing the demand for inferior goods, a rise in income levels will create an increase in the demand for superior goods. In the case of childbearing behaviour, parents with a higher income may not want more children. Instead, they may spend more money per child in order to enhance the quality of their children—just as an increase in income may allow consumers to shift from an economy car to a luxury car. Due to this switch from quantity to quality, a rise in income does not always lead to an increase in the number of children a couple have.

Furthermore, in the New Home Economics theory, the opportunity cost of bearing and rearing children also plays a major role in fertility behavior (Butz and Ward 1979; Mincer 1963). More specifically, having children, even when they are regarded as consumer goods, necessitates a great deal of time being spent on caring for them. Bearing a child and caring for an infant are, in most cases, highly time-intensive activities on the part of mother (assuming a traditional gender role). In particular, since working and childbearing are usually mutually exclusive alternatives for a substantial length of time when women choose to have children, mothers must often give up their gainful occupation during this period. As a result, women are forced to abandon any earnings that could have been obtained in the absence of a child. It therefore follows that a rise in female income, which causes a rise in her opportunity costs, increases the cost of having children relative to other goods and services. This rise will reduce the number of children and result in a fertility decline.

As is the case of fertility, marriage is also regarded as an economic activity in the New Home Economics theory. More specifically, partnership behaviour is delineated through the application of "the principle of comparative advantage" as proposed by the British political economist David Ricardo (1772–1823) (Becker 1973, 1974, 1976; Cigno 1991; Ermisch 2003; Freiden 1974; Oppenheimer 1997; Santos 1975), proceeding upon two basic suppositions. The first of these supposes that men and women allocate their own time to market activity and domestic activity. When engaged in market activity, people work and earn money, whereas people engaged in domestic activity produce "household commodities'" such as meals, good health, washed clothing and children. The consumption of commodities occurs in domestic activity in order to maximize the household's own utility. The second supposition assumes a difference in level between a given man or woman's productivity in market or domestic activities; these differing production capacities in these two different spheres are used as a trade-off in couple formation. Totalizing these assumptions, where men earn a higher wage in the labour market than women, it is assumed that men's efficiency in market activity is relatively superior to that of women. Likewise, when women perform domestic work more efficiently than men, the level of productivity in domestic work is assumed to be higher for women than for men. Based on these two suppositions, Becker and his colleagues regard marriage as a trading process between a man and woman for the maximization of their mutual utility. If, after marriage, one of the partners with a comparative advantage in market production specializes in market work, and the other with a comparative advantage in household production devotes herself or himself to domestic work, then their total utility will become greater and they will be better off by being married than by remaining single. As a result, they will enter into marriage. Conversely, single men and women will not marry and exchange their products with each other if the likely results of their trade-off through marriage are negative with no gain achieved; that is, if each partner perceives that he or she will be worse off by being married than by remaining single. In short, men and women will marry only if it increases their utility. Otherwise, they will remain single. Apparently, this may be regarded as a precise application of the Ricardian principle of comparative advantage.

Easterlin's theory, the latter of the two aforementioned economic theories, also explains marriage and fertility behaviour from a material point of view. According to this theory, relative income determines marriage and childbearing patterns (Easterlin 1961, 1973, 1976, 1978, 1987, 2004; Easterlin et al. 1980; Oppenheimer 1988). To be specific, children who grow to maturity in a cohort with a high standard of living maintain similarly high material expectations as young adults, whereas those who grow up in a cohort with a low standard of living retain low material expectations. Hence, when the present earning potential of young adults is high relative to their material aspirations, their relative economic status is better. In contrast, when the current potential of young adults is low relative to their aspirations, their relative economic status is worse. This status is an index of relative affluence which is defined as a ratio between the earning potential of young people and the level of their material aspirations shaped by their natal household. In many cases, the job opportunities or wage rates of young adults in the labour market are used as the numerator of this ratio, while its denominator is measured by their living standards as children in their parental home.

Based on these assumptions, Easterlin's theory explains demographic behaviour by utilizing the relative economic status between generations. When the relative economic status of young adults is better, they will feel less economic pressure, marry earlier and have more children. In contrast, if their relative economic status is worse, they will feel increasing economic stress, marry later and have fewer children. In short, Easterlin's theory holds that relative economic status, which is formulated by economic and material conditions, determines the patterns of marriage and childbearing.

At first glace, the New Home Economics theory and Easterlin's theory formulate demographic behaviour differently, but they have a fundamental theoretical character in common in that both theories postulate that people's decisions on getting married and having children are made from an economic and materialistic point of view. If entering a married status is economically profitable to both parties, they choose to marry. Likewise, if economic circumstances such as incomes and opportunity costs are favourable for having children, people will become parents. Moreover, when relative economic status is relatively better, young adults get married and have children. Examining the similar characteristics of these two theories, we can clearly see that both the New Home Economics and Easterlin's theories pay almost no attention to the subjective and psychological aspects entailing partnership and parenthood in one's life. The two theories' absence of focus on these areas contrasts strikingly with the attention they are given in the ideational theory. As we will argue in the following section, the ideational theory holds that marriage and fertility behaviour are oriented towards beliefs and values. In the two economic theories discussed, however, such subjective elements are beyond consideration. All in all, both New Home Economics theory and Easterlin's theory insist that changes in the patterns of partnership and childbearing are ultimately attributable to economic conditions in developed countries.

2.4 Second Demographic Transition as Ideational Theory

As discussed above, in the economic theories, objective and material factors play a key role in explaining marriage and reproductive behaviour. In contrast, these demographic behaviours are primarily explained from the viewpoint of ideational and attitudinal factors in the notion of the SDT. Accordingly, instead of seeing marriage and fertility patterns as a consequence of economic conditions such as cost and income, a transformation in partnership and parenthood in developed countries is related to subjective and motivational factors such as values and attitudes (Aassve et al. 2013; Jayakody et al. 2008; Lesthaeghe 1983, 2002; Lesthaeghe and Surkyn 1988; van de Kaa 2001). Due to this characteristic, this explanation is called the ideational theory.

In demographic literature, the importance of ideational or attitudinal factors in marriage and fertility behaviour has never been ignored. For instance, Notestein (1953) already refers to the relation between demographic patterns and the change of social norms and values associated with the process of modernization. Similarly, Hawthorn (1970) emphasizes the importance of subjective factors as determinants of fertility. Moreover, it is also maintained that the process of family formation are not entirely dominated by economic cost–benefit calculations (Murphy 1992; Pollak and Watkins 1993). For instance, based on the comparative analyses of the demographic data obtained from the World Fertility Survey, Cleland and Wilson (1987) find that a fertility decline in less developed countries was more closely associated with parents' cultural factors, such as their new ideas on children, rather than with economic factors such as men's real wages and women's employment. Moreover, Blake (1968) provides a harsh criticism of the notion of children as consumer goods. Indeed, it is pointed out that, even in a contemporary society, children have more functions than giving pleasure (Friedman et al. 1999;

Nauck 2007, 2014; Trommsodorff and Nauck 2005). For instance, having children may consolidate the feeling of solidarity among family members. Such inherent values challenge the notion of children as consumer goods. The historical evidence also suggests that subjective advantages must outweigh disadvantages for a new form of demographic behaviour to emerge (Coale and Watkins 1986). For example, in the First Demographic Transition (FDT) in Europe, which occurred towards the end of the nineteenth century, economic factors alone do not serve to explain the movements of fertility to a satisfactory degree (Lesthaeghe and Wilson 1986). Rather, the findings of the European Fertility Project, which analysed the process of the FDT in Europe, show that the decline in fertility occurred under strikingly diverse socio-economic conditions, and cultural settings had a strong influence on the onset and spread of fertility decline (Coale and Watkins 1986; Knodel and van de Walle 1979; Watkins 1989). For instance, in the case of Belgium, two different linguistic regions under similar economic conditions—i.e., French-speaking Wallonia and Flemish-speaking Fanders—underwent different movements of fertility in the course of the transition (Lesthaeghe 1977), although the European Fertility Project was not designed to examine the effect of culture on reproductive behaviour precisely (Alther 1992). Furthermore, studies of Britain and Germany suggest that variables indicating the level of secularization played an important role in the decline of fertility (Knodel 1974; Teitelbaum 1984). These studies, albeit in their own terminology, reveal in common that subjective and psychological factors play a crucial role in demographic behaviour. Yet, it is since the advocacy of the SDT by Dirk van de Kaa and Ron Lesthaeghe that ideational and attitudinal factors have attracted greater attention in the explanation of partnership and childbearing patterns in developed countries after the 1960s.

Features in the values and attitudes affecting marriage and fertility patterns find interpretive expression in a variety of terms. Examples include the "spread of secular individualism" (Lesthaeghe 1983, 1992, 1995; Lesthaeghe and Meekers 1986; Lesthaeghe and Surkyn 1988), the "advent of adult (or couple)-oriented society" (Ariès 1980), the "increase of progressiveness" (van de Kaa 1980, 1987) or a "move from fundamentalism to pragmatism" (Simons 1982, 1986, 1999). However, these features can be summarized into two points. The first point is that a strong commitment to individualism has manifested itself in developed society, kindling a preoccupation with the pursuit of own goals or the aspiration of self-fulfilment in a social sphere rather than in a domestic sphere. As argued by Maslow (1970), human desires and needs evolve hand in hand with an increase in the level of affluence and security in society. In an earlier stage of economic development, the desire to satisfy material needs ("lower-order needs") have the highest value, because sustenance for existence is relatively scarce. Yet, as a society becomes affluent, the individual priority of needs shifts to personal self-fulfilment ("higher-order needs"), for people do not have to worry about the scarcity of sustenance (Moors and Vermunt 2007). Furthermore, this change has an impact on the pattern of human behaviour in various ways (Inglehart 1977, 1990; Inglehart and Baker 2000; Inglehart and Welzel 2005). As for partnership and family formations, as more weight is placed on individual self-fulfilment within the social sphere, people prefer to pursue their own goals rather than entering into married status or becoming parents (Buchmann 1989; Preston 1986). In short, the ideational theory regards this self-oriented and goal-pursuing attitude as one of the driving forces behind the transformation of partnership and fertility patterns in developed countries.

The second point is that conventional values regulating individual behaviour have weakened, thereby allowing more diverse lifestyles to be accepted. As is argued by by Anthony Wrigley (1978), since major aspects of preindustrial human behaviour were greatly regulated by social norms and institutional control, an individual's family-building process was under the strong influence of so-called traditional values. In other words, individual demographic behaviour was dominated by the "collective consciousness" of a human group (Durkheim 1995). This strong influence was, as a whole, suited to a less developed society where the availability of limited socio-economic resources was threatened by behaviour that deviated from social norms, consequently putting the population's existence at risk (Inglehart 1990; Wrigley 1978). Hence, individual demographic behaviour had to conform to conventional values and customs. In other words, the placement of tight controls on demographic behaviour made it possible for a band of human beings to allocate its relatively scarce resources in an optimal way, securing its continuing existence. Yet, thanks to a high productive capability and material security, demographic behaviour no longer needs to be regulated by traditional norms and values. Consequently, a more tolerant attitude to various types of demographic behaviour is allowed to develop. To put it another way, the regulation mechanism which was upheld by conventional customs and norms tends to give way to the principle of individual free choice in an affluent society and the development of a consciousness that accepts pluralism and diversity. As a result of this change, diverse demographic behaviour such as cohabitation, same-sex marriage and voluntary childlessness, which were rarely seen in the past, are being met with increasing tolerance and acceptance in contemporary society (Lesthaeghe and Meekers 1986; van de Kaa 1987).

Although there is room for further investigation regarding the extent to which these attitudinal changes can account for actual patterns of marriage and fertility, the theoretical framework maintained by the ideational theory is worth noting, for human action is directed by beliefs and values. Looking from the sociological theory of action, human behaviour is guided by the meanings and interpretations ascribed to a person's actions. Specific actions a person takes, at the same time, give meanings and reasons for everyday life. This discursive process can be regarded as a necessary element in the production and reproduction of our conduct (Elster 1986; Garfinkel 1984; Giddens 1979, 1993; Schutz 1943, 1967, 1970). In short, the interpretation of one's actions is affected by the beliefs and values which the actor himself or herself holds, and one's choice of action is made through a process of self-interpretation. Moreover, expressed in terms such as "liquid modernity" and "reflective modernity" (Bauman 2000; Beck et al. 1994; Buchmann 1989; Giddens 1990; Luhmann 1998), self-interpretation of an individual's own behaviour has become more significant than ever in contemporary society. In other words, meanings and accountability in choosing an action become especially important in the process of partnership formation and family building in a contemporary society where the grip of more conventional and institutional elements of family life have weakened (Beck and Beck-Gernsheim 1995; Beck-Gernsheim 2002; Cherlin 2006). Hence, there is no reason to deny that ideational and preferential factors play a crucial role in recent demographic phenomena (Hakim 2003a, b). In fact, it is found that subjective benefits play a key role both in the formation of partnership and in the transition to parenthood (Bernhardt and Goldscheider 2006; Liefbroer 2005; Sobotka 2008a, b; Thornton et al. 2007). Thus, the theoretical framework proposed by the SDT may have enough potentiality for explaining the processes of marriage and fertility behaviour in our affluent world. At the same time, from a viewpoint of scholarly research, we can argue that more significance should be placed on theoretical rather than descriptive aspects in the concept of the SDT.

2.5 Demographic Behaviour as a Purposive Action

As has been already discussed, the economic and the ideational theories provide diverging explanations of marriage and fertility behaviour. The former theory looks at marriage and childbirth from a material and objective point of view; the latter theory examines them through values and attitudes. This contrast is derived from the factors which each theory employs in its explanations, but it is, at the same time, related to the distinct model of human behaviour inherent in each theory. As discussed in a previous section, the characteristics of a given human behavioural model hinge considerably on the way in which reality is abstracted in them (Lindenberg 1992). In other words, the economic and ideational theories are constructed around disparate methodological and epistemological frameworks for marriage and fertility behaviour. Thus, in order to understand the differences between the two theories distinctly, it is necessary to clarify the methodological and epistemological postulates of their behavioural models. We will, in the present section, compare and contrast the behavioural models of these two theories.

When it comes down to the economic theory, its model of a human action is based on two presumptions. First of all, an actor's preferences are stable and exogenously given in the economic model. Indeed, Stigler and Becker (1977) clearly maintain that neoclassical economics should treat human preferences as fixed and exogenous. Accordingly, the extent to which marriage and children bring utility (satisfaction) to people is pre-emptively and transcendentally determined. Second, in the economic theory the purpose of an action is to optimally allocate limited social resources such as wages and time in order to maximize utility with available means. In other words, a human action is taken in order to achieve the utmost satisfaction at the minimum cost which is convertible to monetary terms. Given these premises, it follows that marriage and childbearing occur if they bring more benefits than costs (Blossfeld and Prein 1998). In short, getting married and having children can be regarded as a result of utility-maximizing behaviour with the optimal investment of restricted social resources such as money, time and human capital. Hence, a cost–benefit calculation plays a central role in deciding whether to marry and to have children. Furthermore, if different demographic patterns occur, their causes will be attributable to changes in costs and benefits that marriage and children have brought. For instance, an increase in wages, human capital and opportunity cost may raise a relative cost entailed by entering married status and having children, leading to delayed marriage and fertility decline. This is the behavioural model of the human being according to the economic theory; this is the so-called *homo oekonomicus*.

By contrast, the ideational theory postulates a preference-centred heuristic model of human behaviour (Lindenberg 1991). In other words, human actions are, in this model, directed and motivated by the beliefs and values an actor holds. Hence, the pattern of preference commands an important position in deciding upon an action to be taken. On the methodological side, this behavioural model is constructed on the basis of two presuppositions. First, as in the case of the economic theory, the goal of an action is to maximize satisfaction as determined by an actor's preference. In the ideational theory, however, one's preference is neither fixed nor transcendentally given. One's preference is ceaselessly modified and reformulated by subjective meanings and discursive interpretations of one's conduct. Accordingly, one's preference for getting marriage and having children is neither determined a priori nor fixed. Rather, since one's preference depends on one's own interpretation and meaning-giving, it can be regarded as endogenous and reflective. Second, in the ideational theory, individual beliefs and values affect the subjective meanings and discursive interpretations of human conduct, which consequently sets the desirable and preferable goal of the action. In other words, the purpose to be pursued and the action to be taken depend on individual beliefs and values. Hence, we can argue that beliefs and values play the most crucial role in the choice of an action. Following on with this behavioural model, the advent of new partnership and childbearing behaviours are derived from a change in values and attitudes (Etzioni 1999).

Although the two theories have a different methodological and epistemological framework, it is noteworthy that both of them see demographic behaviour as a purposive action. The two theories also share the view that marriage and fertility behaviour are performed in order to achieve certain goals. As argued by James Coleman (1986, 1990), when human conduct is purposive and goal-directed, it can be regarded as "rational". Moreover, since appropriateness for what an actor attempts to accomplish is central to being rational, a rational action denotes a type of conduct appropriate to achieving the actor's purposes, under given conditions and constraints (Simon 1983). From this point of view, the disparate behavioural models for these two theories can nevertheless be included in a category of rational action (de Bruijn 1999), for the ultimate purpose of a human action is, in the both models, to attain a desirable and preferable goal. In this regard, there is no marked difference between the two behavioural models.

On the other hand, the two theories differ sharply when it comes to concepts of behavioural appropriateness. In the economic theory, an action is appropriate if it can attain a goal with the least amount of economic cost under given constraints (Simon 1978, 1979). In other words, this theory defines a rational action as an action that brings the maximum amount of satisfaction with the minimum expense of social resources. In short, appropriateness of behaviour is seen here to be almost synonymous with means–ends efficacy (Elster 1986). Hence, according to the economic theory, by adhering to economically rational behaviour, one may achieve the optimal allocation of limited means and social resources, under a given constraint (Arrow 1987; Friedman and Hechter 1988; Hogarth and Reder 1987). Values and preference do not play an active role in this theory's working definition of "rational".

By contrast, in the ideational theory, appropriateness of behaviour stands within the realm of an actor's recognition and understanding. More specifically, an action can be seen as rational as long as it achieves what accords with one's beliefs and values. In other words, rationality is immanent in the meaning and interpretation of an action, depending upon the cognitive structure of one's beliefs and values (Simon 1957, 1979, 1987). Thus, if one chooses an action suited to one's beliefs and values, this choice will satisfy the appropriateness of behaviour, and this action will be regarded as rational, regardless of the amount of economic cost involved in goal attaining. We can, therefore, argue that, in the behavioural model of the ideational theory, the criterion of rationality consists in the appropriate link between a value and an action.

When it comes down to a concept of values, many definitions have been put forward in the social science literature so far. For instance, Rokeach (1970) states that a value is a type of belief regarding how one ought to behave or what goal is worth attaining. Similarly, Kluckhohn (1962) claims that a value is a conception of the desirable, which affects the selection of action. Notwithstanding various conceptualizations, it is generally accepted that a value refers to one's enduring belief defined as a desirable (or preferable) mode of conduct or end state (Rokeack 1973). This belief determines the goal to be attained and the action to be taken. Furthermore, when a value is connected to specific objects and situations in an organized way, a specific attitude towards them is cultivated. Hence, a preferable action or end state an individual takes is decided by one's value-orientation. From this point of view, it is natural to think that a preference is neither exogenous nor fixed (Lindenberg 1990). Rather, one's preference is seen as endogenous and changeable. More specifically, one's preference is formed by values in one's belief. Furthermore, if one's beliefs and values change, one's behaviour also transforms in order to accord with one's new preference. Hence, if a change in marriage and fertility behaviour is observed, this is regarded as the outcome of emerging different preferences caused by a shift in values and attitudes.

2.6 Two Types of Rationality in Social Action

As argued above, a marked difference between the two theories exists in the concept of rationality. Rationality in the economic theory is referred to as the material efficacy of means and ends (Heath 1968, 1976). The ideational theory regards rationality as an actor's cognitive and subjective consistency of values and behaviour. We should not forget here that the two types of rationality stand within the long-standing tradition of social action theory (Denzin 1990a, b; Swedberg 1998). It is especially worth noting at this point that Max Weber (1978a, b, 2002) classifies the social actions of human beings into four categories. Weber's first type of the action is an instrumentally rational action, which is taken by the actor with due consideration of conditions and means to attain a goal. The choice to take this action is made if it is the most efficient use of means and resources for the goal-attainment among the other possible uses of them. The instrumentally rational action is goal-oriented in the sense that the goal of the behaviour is determined a priori and the manner in which one behaves is organized only insofar as to choose an optimal means to an end at the minimum expense. The second type of action, according to Weber, is a value-rational action. This action is, regardless of the possible costs, put into practice by an actor's convictions of what is required of him or her by duty, honour, loyalty, faith, ethics, desirability, preference, and so on. Hence, it follows that, when taking the value-rational action, more importance is placed on adherence to a belief in a value and on engagement in a specific behaviour itself than in minimizing costs for the achievement of a goal. The third of Weber's actions is an affectual action, which is inspired by the actor's specific emotional state. This action usually occurs in the form of conscious release of emotional tensions. Weber's forth action is a traditional action, motivated by routine and habit. Traditional action can be seen as an automatic reaction to accustomed stimuli that guide behaviour in a routine course through repetition.

Although this typology of social action is constructed as an ideal type (or pure type), it is, at the same time, useful to understand the economic and the ideational theory from a broader framework of social action. As discussed, one's preference is exogenously given and fixed in the economic theory of marriage and fertility behaviour. Hence, the focal point is how to choose an action that enables the attainment of a goal with optimal means and resources. An actor in the economic theory decides to take a specific action only if it realizes his or her goal with the least amount of cost measurable by a monetary value. This mode of behaviour corresponds to Weber's instrumental rationality. Thus, it follows that, in the economic theory, marriage and fertility behaviour are viewed within a framework of instrumentally rational actions. In the ideational theory, however, since partnership and childbearing behaviour are seen to be guided by beliefs and values, they play a crucial role in choosing an action. In short, the consistent relation between one's values and one's conduct is a key element in the choice of one's actions. This indicates that the behavioural model of the ideational theory can correspond to Weber's value rationality, and marriage and fertility behaviour is viewed within a framework of value-rational action in the ideational theory. Thus, a change in the pattern of partnership and childbearing behaviour in developed countries is explained through instrumental rational choice in the economic theory, whereas it is accounted for through value-rational choice in the ideational theory. From a viewpoint of the social action theory, we can therefore argue that the fundamental difference between the two theories consists in their disparate concepts of rationality.

2.7 The Institutional Environment for Demographic Behaviour

As seen in the previous section, the fundamental difference between behavioural models in the economic and the ideational theory can be found in each theory's concept of rationality. The economic theory is based on instrumental-rational choice, while the ideational theory is constructed around value-rational choice. Thus, when economic factors play an influential role in determining marriage and fertility behaviour in developed countries, it follows that the manner of this behaviour is determined by instrumental rationality. In contrast, where ideational and attitudinal factors are seen to be crucial in determining partnership and family formation, it is safe to say that demographic behaviour is being dominated by value-rationality. It is, however, difficult to determine theoretically which of these two contrasting ideas of rationality plays the dominant role in determining marriage and childbearing behaviour in a specific developed society.

The reason is that institutional settings formally or informally give structural incentives and disincentives to choices of human action, which in turn affect human behaviour and interaction (North 1990, 2005). Human behaviour does not take place in a social vacuum. An institutional environment that includes formal rules, social norms and traditional customs constrains a range of behavioural choices in a society and shapes socially desirable or permissible patterns of human conduct. Through an institutional environment, a microsphere of individual actions is linked to the macro-structure of society. Hence, there is no human action that is separated from social structures (Bourdieu 1977, 2005).

As mentioned earlier, the historical experience of the FDT in Europe shows that fertility started to decline under strikingly diverse socio-economic conditions (Coale and Watkins 1986; Knodel 1974; Knodel and van de Walle 1979; Lesthaeghe 1977; Teitelbaum 1984). Admittedly, the European Fertility Project cannot directly examine the effect of institutional factors on reproductive behaviour, but it is certain that this reduction in family size did not occur free from societal constraints. Rather, institutional settings circumscribe a range of behavioural choices within which people make decisions on the number of children they want to have. Although readiness, willingness, and ability are necessary conditions for fertility control, their influence on reproductive behaviour emerges only when they are socially endorsed (Coale 1973; Lesthaeghe and Vanderhoeft 2001).

It is likely that the institutional environment has a similar impact on the process of partnership and family formation in a contemporary society (Morgan and Taylor 2006; Goldscheider et al. 2015). First, in the economic theory, getting married and having children are seen as the exchange and production of goods and services by partners or couples. These activities inevitably entailtransaction costs (Pollak 1985; Williamson1979, 1981). Since human beings do not automatically have the exact information on a space they require for an action to be taken (Simon 1957), they need to bear the costs involved in grasping details of the environment and the surrounding situation before they can be certain that their action can be successfully accomplished. Social action entails the cost of acquiring the necessary information to guarantee that a given action may take place properly and in accordance with accepted procedure. The same thing holds true for marital formation and childrearing. For instance, if a sufficient number of childcare facilities are supplied, parents can easily find a suitable nursery school to harmonize employment and childrearing. In this case, the institutional environment may give a strong incentive to having children, regardless of couple's earning power. By contrast, if searching for a desirable nursery becomes expensive and there is scant provision of childcare services, worse-off people may think that childrearing is particularly burdensome and risky. Furthermore, they may prefer a small family size in order to avert various kinds of risks in a future (McDonald 2002). In such a situation, economic factors may have a relatively stronger impact on fertility behaviour. As is well known, the availability of childcare services is considerably affected by institutional factors such as welfare and family policies (Brodmann et al. 2007; Neyer 2013). Hence, even if parents behave in the instrumentally rational way, it is likely that the influence of economic factors will vary depending on the institutional context.

In the second place, the informal codes of conduct found in social norms and traditional customs regulate individual behaviour in order to establish cooperative and less frictional human interactions in a society. Since people are embedded in social networks and human relations, they produce socially approved roles and forms of behaviour (Bernardi and Klaerner 2014; Casterline 2001; Granovetter 1985). If a member of a social group takes an action that diverges from such social norms, he or she may suffer informal sanctions, for these norms and customs limit the range of behavioural choices one can make. Thus, if individual values and attitudes are in strong conflict with social norms and conventional customs, people may unwillingly modify their value-rational actions or stop choosing them. Where values and attitudes are weakly confronted by social norms and customs, one may dare to perform one's value-rational actions in the face of social pressure. Whichever option is taken, the fact remains that an actor must bear the psychological cost. Perhaps a high cost would cause the actor to hesitate from taking an action, while a low cost might encourage him or her to choose to act. In short, the psychological cost entailed in a value-rational action will depend on the institutional environment, which, in turn, will provide an incentive or a disincentive for a specific action.

The same holds true in the case of marriage and childbearing behaviour. To be specific, a deep conflict between individual values and institutional norms regarding social and family life may make a value-rational actor highly reluctant to get married and have children. The reason for this is that people could not bear the psychological cost and may avert the risk of disrupting their intimate or personal spheres. However, a less abrasive, more harmonious relation between one's values and social norms may produce a state of willingness on the part of the actor to marry and bear children at modest psychological cost. Social norms regarding the division of gender roles are good cases in point. Indeed, it is indicated that the unequal allocation of domestic work between men and women in developed countries has a bearing on their marriage and fertility behaviour (McDonald 2000a, b, 2006, 2013a, b; Mills 2010). In most cases, a considerable amount of housework is put on a wife's shoulders, while her husband does little or no domestic work. Undoubtedly, this unequal division of domestic labour is sustained mainly by social norms and traditional customs (Rindfuss et al. 1999). This situation is psychologically burdensome for women who set their primary arena for self-fulfilment in the workplace, for cognitive dissonance occurs between their reality and the life they desire. It is, indeed, pointed out that Italian and Japanese women suffer a sharp conflict between intra- and extra-familial roles (Bumpass et al. 2009; McDonald 2002). This conflict needs to be resolved by paying psychological coordination costs. For the sake of harmonizing employment and family life, women may strive for equity in the allocation of domestic work against psychological pressures brought about by the social norms. Yet, in the face of powerful social norms, women may modify their life plan instead and pursue an alternative goal, the desire for self-fulfilment in the workplace notwithstanding. Due to perceived obstacles and anticipated impediments, the desirable goal pursued by value rationality is transformed into a viable option (Ajzen 1988, 1991; Ajzen and Klobas 2013; Fishbein and Ajzen 1975). Moreover, as shown in Aesop's fable "The Fox and the Grapes", beliefs and values may be rationalized to harmonize with a feasible action (Elster 1983, 1990). Thus, coping with informal codes of conduct and a host of social pressures, the process of marriage and childrearing entails psychological coordination costs. If these costs are extremely high, value rationality may play a relatively minor role in marriage and fertility behaviour.

In addition, it should be borne in mind that the initial conditions of institutional contexts will vary from society to society; these conditions will, in turn, affect the development of the space in which a social action will be committed in the future (Nelson and Winter 1982). More specifically, since institutional settings provide behavioural incentives and disincentives at the outset, a specific action may be encouraged or discouraged. The repetition of this action may, in turn, consolidate and reproduce the institutional structure and determine the direction of behavioural changes (Garrouste and Ioannides 2001). In short, since initial institutional conditions determine a future situation, the development of human behaviour has path dependence (David 2001). The same may hold true for partnership and fertility behaviour in developed countries. Even if earning power approaches parity between men and women, every developed country may not experience the same decline in marriage. Likewise, if a value shift occurs in the way that Maslow (1970) formulates, there is no guarantee that divorces and extra-marital births will be ubiquitous in areas outside North-western Europe (Surkyn and Lesthaeghe 2004). From a historical point of view, it appears to be likely that the wide variety of institutional contexts will allow families and partnerships in developed countries to evolve into diverse directions (Thornton 2005). Indeed, the traditional distinction in the pattern of family formation proposed by Hajnal (1983) is still maintained in Europe as a divide between strong and weak forms of family (Reher 2004). By the same token, the rate of extra-marital births has kept relatively low in Italy, although it shares a similar socio-economic situation with other European countries (Dalla Zuanna 2004a, b). Likewise, institutional contexts inherent in Japanese society may be related to its postponement of marriage and childbirth (Bumpass et al. 2009; Tsuya and Bumpass 2004). All in all, the impact of economic and ideational factors on marriage and fertility behaviours is affected by the institutional environment of a society. We can therefore conclude that the relevance of the economic and ideational theories in Japan needs to be examined by an empirical study.

2.8 Conclusion

The primary purpose of this chapter was to reconsider the economic and the ideational theories of marriage and fertility behaviour from a viewpoint of social action theory. For this purpose, the descriptive relevance of the SDT in developed countries was, first of all, examined. Next, we compared and contrasted the methodological and epistemological features of the economic and ideational theories. Subsequently, the behavioural models of the two theories were reformulated from a standpoint of rational choice theory. Finally, the importance of the institutional environment was discussed.

With reference to the descriptive relevance of the SDT, developed countries after the 1960s have experienced more diverse demographic changes than envisaged in this theory. Indeed, even though the TPFR reached the below-replacement level, the rate of extra-marital births or cohabitation varied from one country to another. For this reason, it is not appropriate to regard this grand narrative as a universal description of changes in marriage and fertility behaviour in these countries. Historically speaking, the evolution of demographic patterns is not unilinear, but multilinear. With these points in mind, it is quite difficult to provide a universal description on a change in partnership and family formation in developed countries after the 1960s. Moreover, even if such a description is portrayed, an exceptional case will come into existence. We may therefore argue that the conceptional significance of the SDT does not consist in its descriptive side.

The second point of this chapter was to explore how the economic and the ideational theories differ considerably in the explanation of marriage and fertility behaviour. The former theory explains marriage and childbirth behaviour from a material and objective point of view, while the latter theory accounts for them in terms of values and attitudes. Methodologically speaking, this difference between the two theories was derived from their models of human behaviour. In the economic model, the purpose of a human action is to optimally allocate limited social resources such as wages and time in order to maximize satisfaction (utility). Furthermore, the structure of satisfaction is determined by stable and exogenously given preference. Thus, the central issue of this model is the attainment of a goal with the minimum cost. The ideational theory, however, postulates a preference-centred heuristic model of human behaviour. A preference is formulated by subjective meanings and discursive interpretations. Furthermore, individual beliefs and values produce subjective meanings and discursive interpretations, which consequently work to define desirable conduct. Thus, in this behavioural model, one behaves in the way that accords with one's beliefs and values. Furthermore, it is safe to say that the central significance of the SDT is the application of this heuristic model to marriage and fertility behaviour in developed countries.

As the third point of this chapter, we found that, although these two theories have a different behavioural model, they are arranged in an integrated way from a viewpoint of rational choice theory. The behavioural model for the economic theory can be referred to as a Weberian instrumentally rational action, the goal of which is determined a priori; it is organized only to choose an optimal means to an end at minimal expense. In the ideational theory, however, human behaviour is seen from a viewpoint of value-rational action chosen by an actor's convictions of what is required of him or her, regardless of the possible costs entailed. Despite the differences in the two behavioural models, they are categorized within the realm of rational action. We can, therefore, argue that a fundamental difference between the two theories may be found in the type of rationality postulated.

Fourth, this chapter explored the influence of rationality on marriage and childbearing behaviour as contingent upon an institutional environment. Institutional settings affect the amount of transaction costs necessary for partnership and family formations, which, in turn, have a bearing on the economic costs of marriage and childrearing. At the same time, psychological coordination costs are also affected by institutional factors, which consequently alter the influence of value rationality on demographic behaviours. Taking these points into account, it is safe to say that the impact of economic and attitudinal factors varies from one country to another. Empirical research is, therefore, necessary to judge whether more recent marriage and fertility patterns in Japan are affected by economic or attitudinal factors.

References

Aassve, A., Sironi, M., & Bassi, V. (2013). Explaining attitudes towards demographic behaviour. *European Sociological Review, 29*, 316–333.

Ajzen, I. (1988). *Attitude, personality, and behavior*. Chicago: Dorsey Press.

Ajzen, I. (1991). The theory of planned behavior. *Organizational Behavior and Human Decision Processes, 50*, 179–211.

Ajzen, I., & Klobas, J. (2013). Fertility intentions: An approach based on the theory of planned behavior. *Demographic Research, 29*, 203–232.

Alther, G. (1992). Theories of fertility decline: A non-specialist's guide to the current debate. In J. Gillis, L. A. Tilly, & D. Levine (Eds.), *The European experience of declining fertility, 1850–1970: The quiet revolution* (pp. 13–27). Oxford: Basil Blackwell.

Andorka, R. (1978). *The determinants of fertility in advanced societies*. London: Methuen.

Ariès, P. (1980). Two successive motivations for the declining birth rate in the west. *Population and Development Review, 6*, 645–650.

Arrow, K. J. (1987). Rationality of self and others in an economic system. In R. M. Hogarth & M. W. Reder (Eds.), *Rational choice: The contrast between economics and psychology* (pp. 201–215). Chicago: University of Chicago Press.

Bauman, Z. (2000). *Liquid modernity*. Cambridge: Polity Press.

Beck, U., & Beck-Gernsheim, E. (1995). *The normal chaos of love*. Cambridge: Polity Press.

Beck, U., Giddens, A., & Lash, S. (1994). *Reflexive modernization: Politics, tradition and aesthetics in the modern social order*. Cambridge: Polity Press.

Becker, G. S. (1960). An economic analysis of fertility. In Universities-National Bureau Committee for Economic Research (Ed.), *Demographic and Economic Change in Developed Countries* (pp. 209–231). Princeton: Princeton University Press.

Becker, G. S. (1973). A theory of marriage: Part I. *Journal of Political Economy, 81*, 813–846.

Becker, G. S. (1974). A theory of marriage: Part II. *Journal of Political Economy, 82*, S11–S26.

Becker, G. S. (1976). *The economic approach to human behavior*. Chicago: University of Chicago Press.

Becker, G. S. (1991). *A treaties on the family*. Cambridge, Massachusetts: Harvard University Press.

Becker, G. S. (1986). The economic approach to human behavior. In J. Elster (Ed.), *Rational choice* (pp. 108–122). New York: New York University Press.

Becker, G. S. (1996). *Accounting for tastes*. Cambridge, Massachusetts: Harvard University Press.

Becker, G. S., & Barro, R. J. (1988). A Reformulation of the Economic Theory of Fertility. *Quarterly Journal of Econometrics, 103*, 1–25.

Becker, G. S., & Lewis, H. G. (1973). On the interaction between quantity and quality of children. *Journal of Political Economy, 81*, S279–S288.

Beck-Gernsheim, E. (2002). *Reinventing the family: In search of new lifestyles*. Cambridge: Polity Press.

Bernardi, L., & Klaerner, A. (2014). Social networks and fertility. *Demographic Research, 30*, 641–670.

Bernhardt, E. (2004). Is the second demographic transition a useful concept for demography? *The Vienna Yearbook for Population Research, 2004*, 25–28.

Bernhardt, E., Goldscheider, F. (2006). Gender equality, parenthood attitudes, and first births in Sweden. *Vienna Yearbook of Population Research, 2006*, 19–39.

Billari, F. C., Liefbroer, A. C., & Philipov, D. (2006). The postponement of childbearing in Europe: Driving forces and implications. *Vienna Yearbook of Population Research, 2006*, 1–17.

Blake, J. (1968). Are babies consumer durables? A critique of the economic theory of reproductive motivation. *Population Studies, 22*, 5–25.

Blossfeld, H. P., & Prein, G. (1998). The relationship between rational choice theory and large-scale data analysis: Past developments and future perspectives. In H. P. Blossfeld & G. Prein (Eds.), *Rational choice theory and large-scale data analysis* (pp. 3–27). Boulder: Westview Press.

Bourdieu, P. (1977). *Outline of a theory of practice*. Cambridge: Cambridge University Press.

Bourdieu, P. (2005). *The social structures of the economy*. Cambridge: Polity Press.

Brodmann, S., Esping-Andersen, G., & Güell, M. (2007). When fertility is bargained: Second births in Denmark and Spain. *European Sociological Review, 23*, 599–613.

Buchmann, M. (1989). *The script of life in modern society: Entry into adulthood in a changing world*. Chicago: University of Chicago Press.
Bumpass, L. L., Rindfuss, R. R., Choe, M. K., & Tsuya, N. O. (2009). The institutional context of low fertility: The case of Japan. *Asian Population Studies, 5*, 215–235.
Burgess, E. W., & Locke, H. J. (1945). *The family: From institution to companionship*. New York: The American Book Company.
Butz, W., & Ward, M. (1979). The emergence of counter-cyclical US fertility. *American Economic Review, 69*, 318–328.
Caldwell, J. C. (1982). *Theory of fertility decline*. New York: Academic Press.
Caldwell, J. C. (2006). *Demographic transition theory*. Dordrecht: Springer.
Carmichael, G. (2014). Non-marital pregnancy and the second demographic transition in Australia in historical perspective. *Demographic Research, 30*, 609–640.
Casterline, J. B. (Ed.). (2001). *Diffusion processes and fertility transition: Selected perspectives*. Washigton DC: National Academy Press.
Cherlin, A. J. (2006). *Marriage, divorce, remarriage*. Cambridge, Massachusetts: Harvard University Press.
Cigno, A. (1991). *Economics of the family*. Oxford: Oxford University Press.
Cleland, J., & Wilson, C. (1987). Demand theories of the fertility transition: An iconoclastic view. *Population Studies, 41*, 5–30.
Cliquet, R. L. (1991). *The second demographic transition: Fact or fiction?*. Strasbourg: Council of Europe.
Coale, A. J. (1973). The demographic transition reconsidered. In *Proceedings of the International Population Conference, Liège, 1973* (pp. 53–72). Liège: International Union for the Scientific Study of Population.
Coale, A. J., & Watkins, S. C. (Eds.). (1986). *The decline of fertility in Europe*. Princeton: Princeton University Press.
Coleman, J. S. (1986). Social theory, social research, and a theory of action. *American Journal of Sociology, 91*, 1309–1335.
Coleman, J. S. (1990). *Foundations of social theory*. Cambridge: Belknap Press.
Coleman, D. (Ed.). (1996). *Europe's population in the 1990s*. Oxford: Oxford University Press.
Coleman, D. (2004). Why we don't have to believe without doubting in the 'second demographic transition': Some agnostic comments. *Vienna Yearbook of Population Research, 2004*, 11–24.
Dalla Zuanna, G. (2004a). Few children in strong families: Values and low fertility in Italy. *Genus, 60*, 39–70.
Dalla Zuanna, G. (2004b). The banquet of Aeolus: A familistic interpretation of Italy's lowest low fertility. In G. Dalla Zuanna & G. A. Micheli (Eds.), *Strong family and low fertility: A paradox?* (pp. 105–125). New perspectives in interpreting contemporary family and reproductive behaviour: Kluwer Academic Publisher, Dordrecht.
David, P. A. (2001). Path dependence, its critics, and the quest for 'historical economics'. In P. Garrouste & S. Ioannides (Eds.), *Evolution and path dependence in economic ideas: Past and present* (pp. 15–40). Cheltenham: Edward Elgar.
Davis, K. (1945). The world demographic transition. *Annals of the American Academy of Political and Social Science, 237*, 1–11.
de Bruijn, B. J. (1999). *Foundations of demographic theory: Choice, process, context*. Amsterdam: Thela Thesis.
Demeny, P. (1997). Replacement-level fertility: The implausible endpoint of the demographic transition. In G. W. Jones, R. M. Douglas, J. C. Caldwell, & R. M. D'Souza (Eds.), *The continuing demographic transition* (pp. 94–110). Oxford: Clarendon Press.
Denzin, N. K. (1990a). Reading rational choice theory. *Rationality and Society, 2*, 172–189.
Denzin, N. K. (1990b). The long good-bye: Farewell to rational choice theory. *Rationality and Society, 2*, 504–507.
Duesenberry, J. S. (1960). Comment on Becker's 'an economic analysis of fertility'. In A. J. Coale (Ed.), *Demographic and economic changes in developed countries* (pp. 231–234). Princeton: Princeton University Press.

Durkheim, É. (1995). *The elementary forms of religious life*. New York: Free Press.
Easterlin, R. A. (1961). The American baby boom in historical perspective. *American Economic Review, 51*, 869–911.
Easterlin, R. A. (1973). Relative economic status and the American fertility swing. In E. B. Sheldon (Ed.), *Family economic behavior: Problems and prospects* (pp. 170–223). Philadelphia: J.B. Lippincott.
Easterlin, R. A. (1976). The conflict between aspirations and resources. *Population and Development Review, 2*, 417–425.
Easterlin, R. A. (1978). The economics and sociology of fertility. In C. Tilly (Ed.), *Historical studies of changing fertility* (pp. 57–134). Princeton: Princeton University Press.
Easterlin, R. A. (1987). *Birth and fortune*. Chicago: University of Chicago Press.
Easterlin, R. A. (2004). *The reluctant economist: Perspectives on economics, economic history, and demography*. Cambridge: Cambridge University Press.
Easterlin, R. A., Pollak, R. A., & Wachter, M. L. (1980). Toward a more general economic model of fertility determination: Endogenous preference and natural fertility. In R. A. Easterlin (Ed.), *Population and Economic Change in Developing Countries* (pp. 81–149). Chicago: University of Chicago Press.
Elster, J. (1983). *Sour grapes: Studies in the subversion of rationality*. Cambridge: Cambridge University Press.
Elster, J. (Ed.). (1986). *Rational choice*. New York: New York University Press.
Elster, J. (1990). When rationality fails. In K. S. Cook & M. Levi (Eds.), *The limits of rationality* (pp. 19–51). Chicago: University of Chicago Press.
Ermisch, J. (2003). *An economic analysis of the family*. Princeton: Princeton University Press.
Esteve, A., Lesthaeghe, R., & López-Gay, A. (2012). The latin American cohabitation boom, 1970–2007. *Population and Development Review, 38*, 55–81.
Etzioni, A. (1999). *Essays in socio-economics*. Berlin: Springer.
Fishbein, M., & Ajzen, I. (1975). *Belief, attitude, intention, and behavior: An introduction to theory and research. Reading*. Massachusetts: Addison-Wesley.
Folbre, N. (Ed.). (1996). *The economics of the family*. Cheltenham: Edward Elgar.
Freiden, A. (1974). The United States marriage market. *The Journal of Political Economy, 82*, S34–S53.
Frejka, T., & Sobotka, T. (2008). Fertility in Europe: Diverse, delayed and below replacement. *Demographic Research, 19*, 15–46.
Friedman, D., & Hechter, M. (1988). The contribution of rational choice theory to macrosociological research. *Sociological Theory, 6*, 201–218.
Friedman, D., Hechter, M., & Kanazawa, S. (1999). Theories of the value of children: A new approach. In R. Leete (Ed.), *Dynamics of values in fertility change* (pp. 19–47). Oxford: Oxford University Press.
Garfinkel, H. (1984). *Studies in ethnomethodology*. Cambridge: Polity Press.
Garrouste, P., & Ioannides, S. (Eds.). (2001). *Evolution and path dependence in economic ideas: Past and present*. Cheltenham: Edward Elgar.
Giddens, A. (1979). *Central problems in social theory: Action, structure and contradiction in social analysis*. London: Macmillan Press.
Giddens, A. (1990). *The consequences of modernity*. Cambridge: Polity Press.
Giddens, A. (1993). *New rules of sociological method: A positive critique of interpretative sociologies*. Cambridge: Polity Press.
Goldscheider, F., Bernhardt, E., & Lappegård, T. (2015). The gender revolution: A framework for understanding changing family and demographic behavior. *Population and Development Review, 41*, 207–239.
Goldstein, J. R., Sobotka, T., & Jasilioniene, A. (2009). The end of "lowest-low" fertility? *Population and Development Review, 35*, 663–699.
Granovetter, M. (1985). Economic action and social structure: The problem of embeddedness. *American Journal of Sociology, 91*, 481–510.

Hajnal, J. (1983). Two kinds of pre-industrial household formation system. In R. Wall, J. Robin, & P. Laslett (Eds.), *Family forms in historic Europe* (pp. 65–104). Cambridge: Cambridge University Press.

Hakim, C. (2003a). *Work-lifestyle choices in the 21st century*. Oxford: Oxford University Press.

Hakim, C. (2003b). Preference theory: A new approach to explaining fertility patterns. *Population and Development Review, 29*, 349–374.

Hawthorn, G. (1970). *The sociology of fertility*. London: Collier-MacMillan Ltd.

Heath, A. (1968). Economic theory and sociology. *Sociology, 2*, 273–292.

Heath, A. (1976). *Rational choice and social exchange: A critique of exchange theory*. Cambridge: Cambridge University Press.

Henrich, J., Boyd, R., Bowles, S., Camerer, C., Fehr, E., & Gintis, H. (Eds.). (2004). *Foundations of human sociality: Economic experiments and ethnographic evidence from fifteen small-scale societies*. Oxford: Oxford University Press.

Hogarth, R. M., & Reder, M. W. (Eds.). (1987). *Rational choice: The contrast between economics and psychology*. Chicago: University of Chicago Press.

Iacovou, M., & Parisi, L. (2009). Leaving home. In M. Brynin & J. Ermisch (Eds.), *Changing relationships* (pp. 59–72). New York: Routledge.

Inglehart, R. (1977). *The silent revolution: Changing values and political styles among western publics*. Princeton: Princeton University Press.

Inglehart, R. (1990). *Culture shift in advanced industrial society*. Princeton: Princeton University Press.

Inglehart, R., & Baker, W. E. (2000). Modernization, cultural change, and the persistence of traditional values. *American Sociological Review, 65*, 19–51.

Inglehart, R., & Welzel, C. (2005). *Modernization, cultural change, and democracy: The human development sequence*. Cambridge: Cambridge University Press.

Jayakody, R., Thornton, A., & Axinn, W. (Eds.). (2008). *International family change: Ideational perspectives*. New York: Lawrence Erlbaum Associates.

Kiernan, K. (1996). Partnership behaviour in Europe: Recent trends and issues. In D. Coleman (Ed.), *Europe's population in the 1990s* (pp. 62–91). Oxford: Oxford University Press.

Kiernan, K. (1999a). Cohabitation in Western Europe. *Population Trends, 96*, 23–32.

Kiernan, K. (1999b). Childbearing outside marriage in Western Europe. *Population Trends, 98*, 11–20.

Kiernan, K. (2001). The rise of cohabitation and childbearing outside marriage in Western Europe. *International Law, Policy and the Family, 15*, 1–21.

Kiernan, K. (2004). Unmarried cohabitation and parenthood in Britain and Europe. *Journal of Law and Policy, 26*, 33–55.

Kluckhohn, C. (1962). Values and value-orientation in the theory of action. In T. Parsons & E. A. Shils (Eds.), *Toward a general theory of action* (pp. 388–433). New York: Harper & Row.

Knodel, J. (1974). *The decline of fertility in Germany, 1871–1939*. Princeton: Princeton University Press.

Knodel, J., & van de Walle, E. (1979). Lessons from the past: Policy implications of historical fertility studies. *Population and Development Review, 5*, 217–245.

Kohler, H. P., Billari, F. C., & Ortega, J. A. (2002). The emergence of lowest-low fertility in Europe during the 1990s. *Population and Development Review, 28*, 641–680.

Kreager, P. (2015). Population theory: A long view. *Population Studies, 69*, S29–S37.

Leibenstein, H. (1974). Socio-economic fertility theories and their relevance to population policy. *International Labour Review, 109*, 443–457.

Leibenstein, H. (1975). The economic theory of fertility decline. *Quarterly Journal of Economics, 89*, 1–31.

Leibenstein, H. (1976). *Beyond economic man: A new foundation for microeconomics*. Cambridge, Massachusetts: Harvard University Press.

Leibenstein, H. (1981). Economic decision theory and human fertility behavior: A speculative essay. *Population and Development Review, 7*, 381–400.

Lesthaeghe, R. (1977). *The decline of Belgian fertility, 1800–1970*. Priceton: Princeton University Press.

Lesthaeghe, R. (1983). A century of demographic and cultural change in Western Europe. *Population and Development Review, 9*, 411–436.

Lesthaeghe, R. (1992). Beyond economic reductionism: The transformation of the reproductive regimes in France and Belgium in the 18th and 19th Centuries. In C. Goldscheider (Ed.), *Fertility transitions, family structure, and population policy* (pp. 1–44). Boulder: Westview Press.

Lesthaeghe, R. (1995). The second demographic transition in western countries: An interpretation. In K. O. Mason & A. M. Jensen (Eds.), *Gender and family change in industrialized countries* (pp. 1–18). Oxford: Clarendon Press.

Lesthaeghe, R. (2001). *Postponement and recuperation: Recent fertility trends and forecasts in six Western European Countries*. Interuniversity Papers in Demography. Gent: Universiteit Gent.

Lesthaeghe, R. (2002). *Meaning and choice: Value orientations and life course decision*. The Hague: NIDI CBGS Publications.

Lesthaeghe, R. (2010). The unfolding story of the second demographic transition. *Population and Development Review, 36*, 211–251.

Lesthaeghe, R. (2014). The second demographic transition: A concise overview of its development. *Proceedings of the National Academy of Sciences, 111*, 18112–18115.

Lesthaeghe, R., & Meekers, D. (1986). Value changes and the dimension of familism in the European community. *European Journal of Population, 2*, 225–268.

Lesthaeghe, R., & Permanyer, I. (2014). *European sub-replacement fertility: Trapped or recovering?*. Ann Arbor: Population Studies Center, University of Michigan.

Lesthaeghe, R., & Surkyn, J. (1988). Cultural dynamics and economic theories of fertility change. *Population and Development Review, 14*, 1–45.

Lesthaeghe, R., & Vanderhoeft, C. (2001). Ready, willing, and able: A conceptualization of transitions to new behavioral forms. In J. B. Casterline (Ed.), *Diffusion processes and fertility transition* (pp. 240–264). Washington, D.C.: National Academy Press.

Lesthaeghe, R., & Willems, P. (1999). Is low fertility a temporary phenomenon in the European Union? *Population and Development Review, 25*, 211–228.

Lesthaeghe, R., & Wilson, C. (1986). Modes of production, secularization and the pace of the fertility decline in Western Europe, 1870–1930. In A. J. Coale & S. C. Watkins (Eds.), *The decline of fertility in Europe* (pp. 261–292). Princeton: Princeton University Press.

Levy, M. J. (1966). *Modernization and the structure of societies: A setting for international affairs*. Princeton: Princeton University Press.

Liefbroer, A. C. (2005). The impact of perceived costs and rewards of childbearing on entry into parenthood: Evidence from a panel study. *European Journal of Population, 21*, 367–391.

Lindenberg, S. (1990). Home Socio-oeconomicus: The emergence of a general model of man in the social sciences. *Journal of Institutional and Theoretical Economics, 146*, 727–748.

Lindenberg, S. (1991). Social approval, fertility and female labour market. In J. J. Siegers, J. de Jong-Gierveld, & E. van Imhoff (Eds.), *Female labour market behaviour and fertility: A rational-choice approach* (pp. 32–58). Berlin: Springer.

Lindenberg, S. (1992). The method of decreasing abstraction. In J. S. Coleman & T. J. Fararo (Eds.), *Rational choice theory: Advocacy and critique* (pp. 3–20). Newbury Park: Sage Publications.

Luhmann, N. (1998). *Observations on modernity*. Stanford: Stanford University Press.

Maslow, A. H. (1970). *Motivation and personality*. New York: Harper & Row.

McDonald, P. (2000a). Gender equity in theories of fertility transition. *Population and Development Review, 26*, 427–439.

McDonald, P. (2000b). Gender equity, social institutions and the future of fertility. *Journal of Population Research, 17*, 1–16.

McDonald, P. (2002). Sustaining fertility through public policy: The range of options. *Population (English Edition), 57*, 417–446.

McDonald, P. (2006). Low fertility and the state: The efficacy of policy. *Population and Development Review, 32*, 485–510.
McDonald, P. (2013a). Societal foundations for explaining fertility: Gender equity. *Demographic Research, 28*, 981–994.
McDonald, P. (2013b). Challenges for European family and fertility research. In G. Neyer, G. Andersson, H. Kulu, L. Bernardi, & C. Bühler (Eds.), *The demography of Europe* (pp. 15–27). Dordrecht: Springer.
McNicoll, G. (1992). The agenda of population studies: A commentary and complaint. *Population and Development Review, 18*, 399–420.
McNicoll, G. (2012). Reflections on post-transition demography. In G. McNicoll, J. Bongaarts, & E. P. Churchill (Eds.), *Population and public policy: Essays in honor of Paul Demeny* (pp. 3–19). New York: The Population Council.
Mills, M. (2010). Gender roles, gender (In)equality and fertility: An empirical test of five gender equity. *Canadian Studies in Population, 37*, 445–474.
Mincer, J. (1963). Market prices, opportunity costs and income effects. In C. F. Christ, M. Friedman, L. A. Goodman, Z. Griliches, A. C. Harberger, N. Liviatan, J. Mincer, Y. Mundlak, M. Nerlove, D. Patinkin, L. G. Telser, & H. Theil (Eds.), *Measurement in econometrics: Studies in mathematical economics and econometrics in memory of Yehuda Grunfeld* (pp. 67–82). Stanford: Stanford University Press.
Moore, W. E. (1974). *Social change*. Englewood Cliffs: Prentice-Hall.
Moors, G., & Vermunt, J. (2007). Heterogeneity in post-materialist value priorities: Evidence from a latent class discrete choice approach. *European Sociological Review, 2*, 631–648.
Morgan, S. P., & Taylor, M. G. (2006). Low fertility at the turn of the twenty-first century. *Annual Review of Sociology, 32*, 375–399.
Murphy, M. (1992). Economic models of fertility in post-war Britain: A conceptual and statistical re-interpretation. *Population Studies, 46*, 235–258.
Nauck, B. (2007). Value of children and the framing of fertility: Results from a cross-cultural comparative survey in 10 societies. *European Sociological Review, 23*, 615–629.
Nauck, B. (2014). Value of children and the social production of welfare. *Demographic Research, 30*, 1793–1824.
Nelson, R. R., & Winter, S. G. (1982). *An evolutionary theory of economic change*. Cambridge, Massachusetts: Harvard University Press.
Neyer, G. (2013). Welfare states, family policies, and fertility in Europe. In G. Neyer, G. Andersson, H. Kulu, L. Bernardi, & C. Bühler (Eds.), *The demography of Europe* (pp. 29–53). Dordrecht: Springer.
Ní Bhrolcháin, M., & Beaujouan, É. (2013). Education and cohabitation in Britain: A return to traditional patterns? *Population and Development Review, 39*, 441–458.
North, D. C. (1990). *Institutions, institutional change and economic performance*. Cambridge: Cambridge University Press.
North, D. C. (2005). *Understanding the process of economic change*. Princeton: Princeton University Press.
Notestein, F. W. (1953). Economic problems of population change. In *Proceedings of the Eighth International Conference of Agricultural Economists* (pp. 13–31). Oxford: Oxford University Press.
Ogburn, W. F., & Nimkoff, M. F. (1955). *Technology and the changing family*. Boston: Houghton Mifflin Company.
Oppenheimer, V. K. (1988). A theory of marriage timing. *American Journal of Sociology, 94*, 563–591.
Oppenheimer, V. K. (1997). Women's employment and the gain to marriage: The specialization and trading model. *Annual Review of Sociology, 23*, 431–453.
Parsons, T., & Bales, R. F. (Eds.). (1955). *Family, socialization and interaction process*. New York: The Free Press.
Pollak, R. A. (1985). A transaction cost approach to families and households. *Journal of Economic Literature, 23*, 581–608.

Pollak, R. A., & Watkins, S. C. (1993). Cultural and economic approaches to fertility: Proper marriage or Mésalliance? *Population and Development Review, 19*, 467–496.
Potârcă, G., Mills, M., & Lesnard, L. (2013). Family formation trajectories in Romania, the Russian federation and France: Towards the second demographic transition? *European Journal of Population, 29*, 69–101.
Preston, S. H. (1986). Changing values and falling birth rates. In K. Davis, M. S. Bernstam, & R. Ricardo-Campbell (Eds.), *Below-replacement fertility in industrial societies* (pp. 176–195). New York: The Population Council.
Reher, D. S. (2004). Family ties in Western Europe persistent contrasts. In G. Dalla Zuanna & G. A. Micheli (Eds.), (pp. 45–76) Strong family and low fertility: A paradox? New perspectives in interpreting contemporary family and reproductive behaviour. Dordrecht: Kluwer Academic.
Rindfuss, R. R., Brewster, K. L., & Kavee, A. L. (1999). Women, work, and children: Behavioral and ideational change in the United State. In R. Leete (Ed.), *Dynamics of values in fertility change* (pp. 148–175). Oxford: Oxford University Press.
Rokeach, M. (1970). *Beliefs, attitudes, and values*. San Francisco: Jossey-Bass.
Rokeach, M. (1973). *The nature of human values*. New York: The Free Press.
Rosenzweig, M. R., & Stark, O. (Eds.). (1997). *Handbook of population and family economics 1A*. Amsterdam: Elsevier.
Santos, F. P. (1975). The economics of marital status. In C. B. Lloyd (Ed.), *Sex, discrimination, and the division of labor* (pp. 244–269). New York: Columbia University Press.
Schultz, T. W. (Ed.). (1974). *Economics of the family*. Chicago: University of Chicago Press.
Schutz, A. (1943). The problem of rationality in the social world. *Economica, 10*, 130–149.
Schutz, A. (1967). *The phenomenology of social world*. Evanston: Northwestern University Press.
Schutz, A. (1970). *On phenomenology and social relations*. Chicago: University of Chicago Press.
Simon, H. A. (1957). *Models of man: Social and rational*. New York: Wiley.
Simon, H. A. (1978). Rationality as process and as product of thought. *American Economic Review, 68*, 1–16.
Simon, H. A. (1979). From substantive to procedural rationality. In F. Hahn & M. Hollis (Eds.), *Philosophy and economic theory* (pp. 65–86). Oxford: Oxford University Press.
Simon, H. A. (1983). *Models of bounded rationality: Behavioral economics and business organization*. Cambridge, Massachusetts: The MIT Press.
Simon, H. A. (1985). Human nature in politics: The dialogue of psychology with political science. *American Political Science Review, 79*, 239–304.
Simon, H. A. (1987). Rationality in psychology and economics. In R. M. Hogarth & M. W. Reder (Eds.), *Rational choice: The contrast between economics and psychology* (pp. 25–40). Chicago: University of Chicago Press.
Simons, J. (1982). Reproductive behaviour as religious practice. In C. Höhn & R. Mackensen (Eds.), *Determinants of fertility trends: Theories re-examined* (pp. 133–145). Liège: Ordina.
Simons, J. (1986). How conservative are british attitudes to childbearing. *Quarterly Journal of Social Affairs, 2*, 415–429.
Simons, J. (1999). The cultural significance of western fertility trends in the 1980s. In R. Leete (Ed.), *Dynamics of values in fertility change* (pp. 78–99). Oxford: Oxford University Press.
Smelser, N. J. (1959). *Social change in the industrial revolution: An application of theory to the British cotton industry*. Chicago: University of Chicago Press.
Sobotka, T. (2008a). The diverse faces of the second demographic transition in Europe. *Demographic Research, 19*, 171–224.
Sobotka, T. (2008b). Does persistent low fertility threaten the future of European populations? In J. Surkyn, P. Deboosere, & J. Van Bavel (Eds.), *Demographic challenges for the 21st century: A state of the art in demography* (pp. 27–89). Brussels: VUBPRESS.
Stigler, G. J., & Becker, G. S. (1977). De Gustibus Non Est Disputandum. *The American Economic Review, 67*, 76–90.

Surkyn, J., & Lesthaeghe, R. (2004). Value orientations and the second demographic transition (SDT) in Northern, Western and Southern Europe: An update. *Demographic Research, 3*, 45–86.
Swedberg, R. (1998). Max Weber's vision of economic sociology. *The Journal of Socio-Economics, 27*, 473–574.
Teitelbaum, M. S. (1984). *The British fertility decline*. Princeton: Princeton University Press.
Thompson, W. S. (1929). Population. *American Journal of Sociology, 34*, 959–975.
Thornton, A. (2005). *Reading history sideways: The fallacy and enduring impact on the developmental paradigm on family life*. Chicago: University of Chicago Press.
Thornton, A., Axinn, W. G., & Xie, Y. (2007). *Marriage and cohabitation*. Chicago: University of Chicago Press.
Trommsodorff, G., & Nauck, B. (Eds.). (2005). *The value of children in cross-cultural perspective: Case studies from eight societies*. Lengerich: Pabst Science Publishers.
Tsuya, N. O., & Bumpass, L. L. (Eds.). (2004). *Marriage, work, and family life in comparative perspective: Japan, South Korea, and the United States*. Honolulu: University of Hawai'i Press.
van de Kaa, D. J. (1980). Recent trend in fertility in Western Europe. In R. W. Hiorns (Ed.), *Demographic patterns in developed societies* (pp. 55–83). London: Taylor and Francis.
van de Kaa, D. J. (1987) Europe's second demographic transition. *Population Bulletin, 42*.
van de Kaa, D. J. (1994). The second demographic transition revisited: Theories and expectations. In G. Beets (Ed.), *Population and family in the low countries 1993: Late fertility and other current issues* (pp. 81–126). Lisse: Swets & Zeitlinger.
van de Kaa, D. J. (1996). Anchored narratives: The story and findings of half a century of research into the determinants of fertility. *Population Studies, 50*, 389–432.
van de Kaa, D. J. (2001). Postmodern fertility preferences: From changing value orientation to new behaviour. In R. A. Bulatao & J. B. Casterline (Eds.), *Global Fertility Transition* (pp. 290–331). New York: Population Council.
van de Kaa, D. J. (2003). The idea of a second demographic transition in industrialized Countries. *Journal of Population and Social Security, 1*, 1–34.
Watkins, S. C. (1989). The fertility transition: Europe and the third world compared. In J. M. Stycos (Ed.), *Demography as an interdiscipline* (pp. 27–55). New Brunswick: Transaction Publishers.
Weber, M. (1978a). *Economy and society: An outline of interpretive sociology*. Berkeley: University of California Press.
Weber, M. (1978b). The foundations of social theory. In W. B. Runciman (Ed.), *Max Weber selections in translation* (pp. 3–61). Cambridge: Cambridge University Press.
Weber, M. (2002). *Basic concepts in sociology*. New York: Kensington Publishing.
Werding, M. (2014). Children are costly, but raising them may pay: The economic approach to fertility. *Demographic Research, 30*, 253–276.
Williamson, O. E. (1979). Transaction-cost economics: The governance of contractual relations. *Journal of Law and Economics, 22*, 233–261.
Williamson, O. E. (1981). The economics of organization: The transaction cost approach. *American Journal of Sociology, 87*, 548–577.
Willis, R. J. (1973). A new approach to the economic theory of fertility behavior. *Journal of Political Economy, 81*, S14–S64.
Wilson, C. (2013). Thinking about post-transitional demographic regimes: A reflection. *Demographic Research, 28*, 1373–1388.
Wrigley, E. A. (1978). Fertility strategy for the individual and the group. In C. Tilly (Ed.), *Historical studies of changing fertility* (pp. 135–154). Princeton: Princeton University Press.

Chapter 3
Economic Change, Value Shift and Marriage Behaviour

3.1 Introduction

In our present investigation of demographic behaviour in Japan, we will first examine whether Japanese marriage patterns are affected by economic and ideational factors. We will second explore the extent to which the transition from single status to married status has an impact on attitudes towards partnership and family.

As in the case of Japan, marriage patterns have changed over the past few decades across many industrialized countries. To site one example of nuptial change, people are marrying much later in life than has been previously seen. By 2009, male age at first marriage had risen to around 32 years in France and the UK, and 33 years in Italy and Germany. In the same year, women entered into marriage at around their thirtieth birthday in France, the UK, Italy and Germany (see Graph 3.1). In short, developed countries are facing rapid changes in the timing of partnership formation.

Japan is no exception. Marriage has undergone drastic changes in Japan in recent years (Tsuya and Bumpass 2004). The timing of entry into marriage is becoming increasingly delayed; concurrently, bachelors and spinsters are increasing in number. Under these circumstances, it would seem that marriage is losing its appeal; the attractive glow that it once held in Japan is clearly diminishing. For instance, by 2009, the mean age at first marriage had risen to 30.4 years of age for men and 28.6 years for women. Looking at these figures, it becomes clear that changes in marriage patterns are not limited to Western countries; they are also seen in Japan. In addition, these transformations are strongly connected to the low fertility rate in Japan, where extra-marital births are rare and most children are born within wedlock. This being the case, the increasing number of unmarried people and the delay in the timing of marriage serve together to compress the reproductive period and to reduce the number of reproductive units. This consequently leads to a decrease in the number of births.

N. Fukuda, *Marriage and Fertility Behaviour in Japan*,
DOI 10.1007/978-981-10-0294-6_3

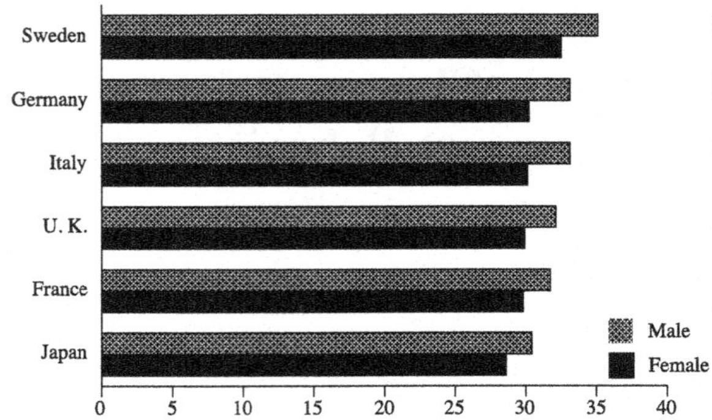

Graph. 3.1 Mean age at first marriage in 2009, selected countries. *Source* UNECE Statistical Database

In this chapter, we will begin by considering salient features of Japanese marriage behaviour. Then, we will discuss the relation between Japanese marriage patterns and societal changes. Thereafter, the determinants of marriage behaviour will be examined, followed by an explanation of data and methods used this analysis. Finally, we will examine the influence of marriage on attitudes towards partnership and family relations.

3.2 Changing Features of Japanese Marriage Patterns

In this section, we will discuss changes in the features of Japanese marriage behaviour. The point to be noted is, first of all, a sharp rise in men's and women's marriage ages. To be specific, the Japanese marriage age did not rise continuously over the post-war period. Looking at the whole period after the Second World War, age at marriage remained quite stable until the end of 1970s (see Graph 3.2). Japanese men, on the average, got married at around age 26, while women entered into a married status at around their 25th birthday. However, marriage age rose rapidly in Japan from the latter half of the 1970s and onwards. In fact, the mean age at first marriage for men rose sharply from 27.0 in 1975 to 30.5 in 2010; for women, first-marriage age also increased, from 24.7 to 28.8, over the same period. It follows that the timing of marriage became delayed by approximately three years over the course of these three decades. Furthermore, it is noteworthy that this rise in marriage age went hand in hand with a fertility decline. As shown in Graph 3.2, the Japanese total period fertility rate (TPFR) remained stable at about two births per woman from 1957 until 1973, except for a dip in 1966, the "Year of the Fire Horse", which has been traditionally considered an unlucky year for giving birth to girls. However, the TPFR started to show a downward trend from the mid-1970s, falling from 2.14 births per woman in 1973 to 1.39 in 2010 in tandem with a rise in marriage age.

The second salient feature in our examination of changes in marriage behaviour is an increase in the numbers of unmarried men and women, which is coincidently

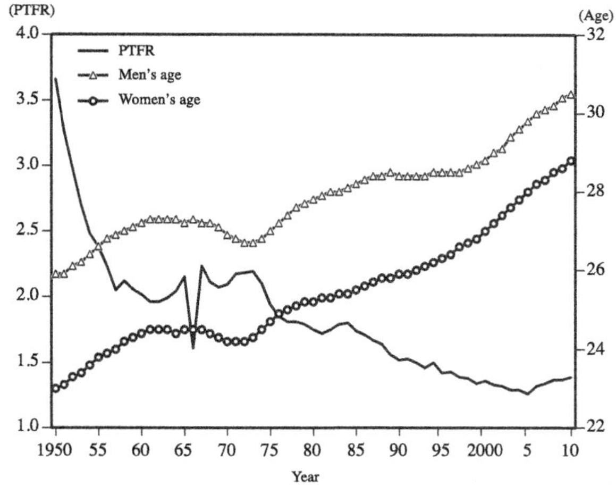

Graph. 3.2 Mean age at first marriage in Japan. *Source* The Ministry of Health, Labour and Welfare (various years). Vital statistics

occurring with the aforementioned delayed entry into married status and increasing lifelong celibacies in number (Raymo 1998; Retherford et al. 2001). Theoretically, a rise in marriage age does not always result in an increase in the proportion of people never-married. For example, if young adults who remained single in their 30s rush to marry in their 40s, they can avoid becoming lifelong celibates. Yet, the postponement of marriage timing is connected to an increase in the proportion of single middle-aged adults in Japan. As clearly shown in Graph 3.3, the proportion of single men and women has steadily increased since 1980. To take an example, the percentage of men aged 50–54 who had never married was only 2.1 % in 1980, whereas the percentage sharply jumped to 17.8 % in 2010. Likewise, the proportion of women never-married in the 50–54 age group also rose steeply from 4.4 % in 1980 to 8.7 % in 2010. According to Brinton (1993), individuals' sense of what is generally felt to be an appropriate time to marry plays a key role in determining marriage decisions in Japanese society. Due to this inflexibility in what is perceived to be appropriate in terms of experiencing life events, Japanese people who do not marry at what they consider to be an appropriate age may remain single for life.

A third pointed shift in marriage behaviour is an increase in the number of marriage dissolution. In fact, divorces have increased in number since the mid-1970s in Japan, and the Japanese divorce rate has now caught up with their European counterparts (Raymo et al. 2004). As shown in Graph 3.4, the crude divorce rate stood at around 2.0 per thousand in Germany, Sweden and the UK in 1975. By contrast, the Japanese rate was relatively low, standing at only 1.07 in 1975. It, however, rose sharply to 1.99 by 2010. France, Germany, Sweden and the UK showed a crude divorce rate of about 2.0 in 2009, so the 2010 Japanese figure does not compare favourably with the European figures; the gap in the divorce rate between Japan and Europe has narrowed considerably.

The fourth feature to be noted is that, compared with North-western Europe, cohabitation is rare in Japan. Cohabitation was broadly chosen as the formation of

Graph. 3.3 The percentage of never-married people in Japan. **a** Men and **b** women. *Source* The Ministry of Internal Affairs and Communications (various years). National Census

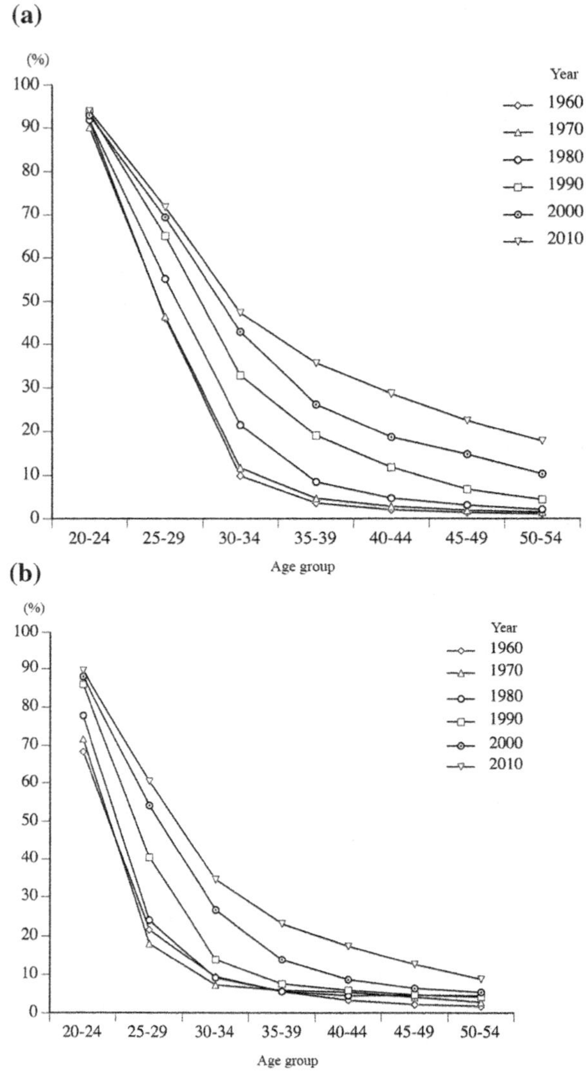

a first union among young adults in North-western Europe in the 1980s, spreading across Mediterranean countries from the late 1990s (Gabrielli and Hoem 2010; Rosina and Fraboni 2004). Likewise, the USA has experienced a marked increase in cohabitation since the 1980s (Smock 2000). Admittedly, as shown in Graph 3.5, the percentages of men and women experiencing cohabitation are showing a steady upward trend in Japan until 2005, although the figures decreased slightly in 2010. For instance, the percentage of men aged 25–29 who had, at some point, experienced cohabitation rose threefold from 3.3 % in 1987 to 11.8 % in 2005. Similarly, the percentage of women ever-cohabited in the 25–29 age group also increased

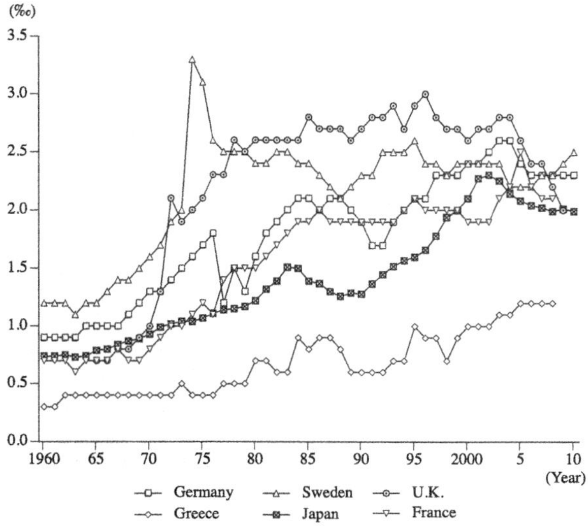

Graph. 3.4 The crude divorce rate from 1960 to 2010, selected countries. *Source* Eurostat Statistical Database

steeply from 4.1 to 10.1 % in the same period. Yet, cohabitation is far less prevalent in Japan than in European countries. In fact, approximately 40 % of men between ages 25 and 29 were cohabiting in Sweden and Norway even in the mid-1990s. Likewise, the percentage of Swedish and Norwegian women aged between 25 and 29 who were cohabiting was above 30 % in the same period (Kiernan 2000, 2001, 2002, 2004a, b). At around the same time, in 1996, the percentage figures in Belgium and the UK stood at 10 % for cohabiting men and women aged 25–29; the cohabitation prevalence figures for Japan in the year 2005 are close to these 1996 British and Belgian figures. Where the spread of cohabitation is concerned, Japan appears to be lagging close to ten years or more behind European countries.

Finally, we need to make reference to pregnancy-dependent marriage as another changing feature of Japanese marriage (Raymo and Iwasawa 2008). The Ministry of Health, Labour and Welfare (2010) defines premarital pregnancy as a first baby to couples who have been legally married for less than 37 weeks. Hence, if a couple had a first child within 37 weeks of marriage, it follows that they entered into married status after the female partner's pregnancy was confirmed. As shown in Graph 3.6, the proportion of marriages involving premarital pregnancy is on the increase. For instance, the percentage of legitimate first births involving premarital pregnancy over the total legitimate first births stood at only 7.8 % for mothers aged 24–29 in 1980, while the figure rose steeply to 24.6 % in 2009. Similarly, 20.1 % of married women between ages 20 and 24 bore their first child as a result of a premarital pregnancy in 1980; this figure jumped to 63.6 % in 2009.

Premarital conceptions may, theoretically, be terminated with induced abortions (Bongaarts and Potter 1983). Yet, as far as Graph 3.7 shows, age-specific abortion rates for young adults have tended to decline over the past few decades, with the exception of a temporal surge in the abortion rate of the under-age group around the year 2000. Hence, it may be that an increase in the proportion

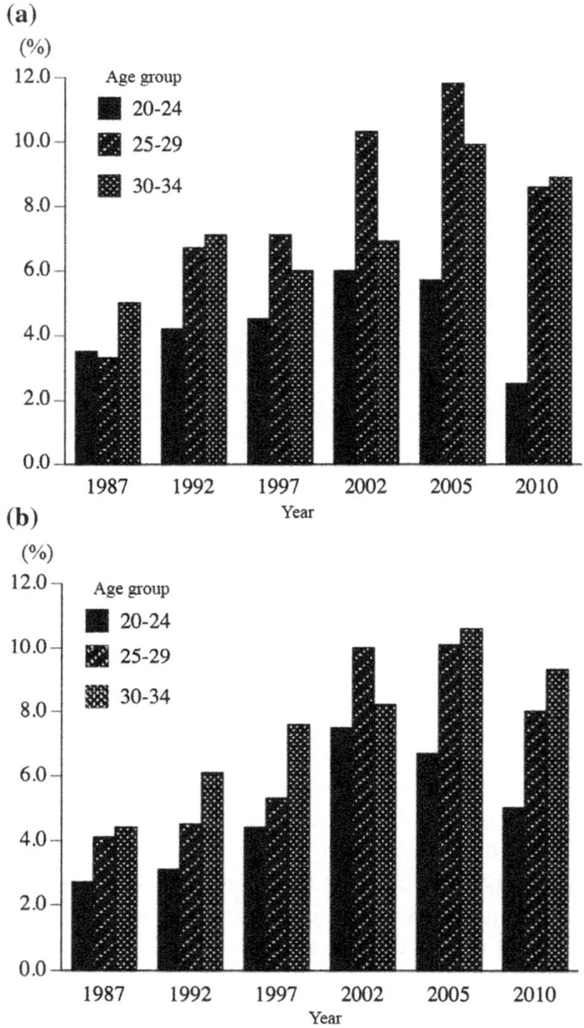

Graph. 3.5 The percentage of people ever-cohabited in Japan. **a** Men and **b** women. *Source* National Institute of Population and Social Security Research (2012). The report on the Fourteenth Japanese National Fertility Survey in 2010

of pregnancy-dependent marriages is related to a reduction in the abortion rate. In other words, we may infer that, once a premarital conception is confirmed, most couples choose to marry rather than to terminate the pregnancy. Taking these points into consideration, we may argue that premarital pregnancy is a trigger for marriage in Japan. In short, unmarried couples may be rushing to enter into a legal marriage when they find they are pregnant.

As discussed above, Japan has experienced radical changes in marriage patterns. The societal mechanisms which have brought about these changes, however, have not been sufficiently clarified. In the following section, we will discuss some of the theories which attempt to explain these changes in marriage behaviour, focusing on socio-economic and ideational aspects.

Graph. 3.6 The percentage of pregnancy-dependent marriages over all marriages in Japan. *Source* The Ministry of Health, Labour and Welfare (2010). The special report on Vital Statistics

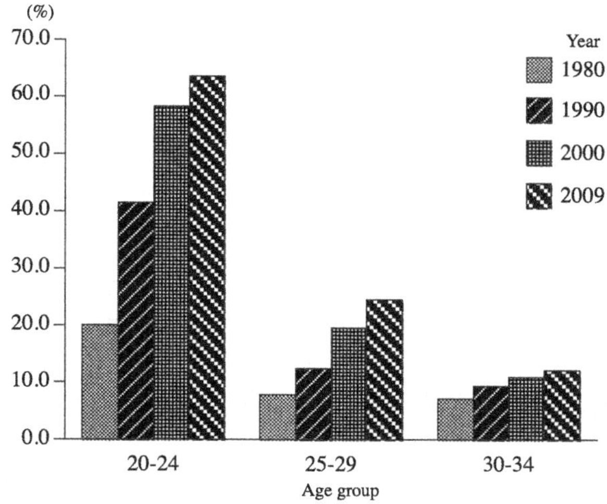

Graph. 3.7 The age-specific induced abortion rate in Japan. *Source* The Ministry of Health, Labour and Welfare (various years). Report on Public Health Administration and Services

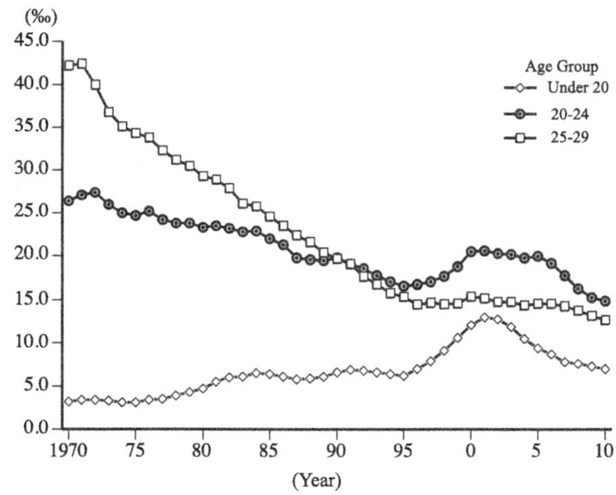

3.3 Economic and Attitudinal Changes in Japan

As mentioned earlier in this chapter, not only Japan but also other developed countries have experienced changes in marriage behaviour, though not necessary to the same degree.[1] Several studies have already been carried out concerning changes in marriage patterns as seen in Western countries[2] (Carter and Glick 1976; Cherline 1992; Cigno 1991; Easterlin 1987; Eldridge and Kiernan 1985; Ermisch 1981, 2003;

[1]For further details of the comparison of marriage and fertility patterns among industrialized countries, see van de Kaa (1987) and Coleman (1993).

[2]For a discussion of the change of marriage patterns in the USA, see Cherline (1992).

Graph. 3.8 Labour participation rate of women aged 20–44 in Japan. *Source* The Ministry of Internal Affairs and Communications (various years). Labour Force Survey

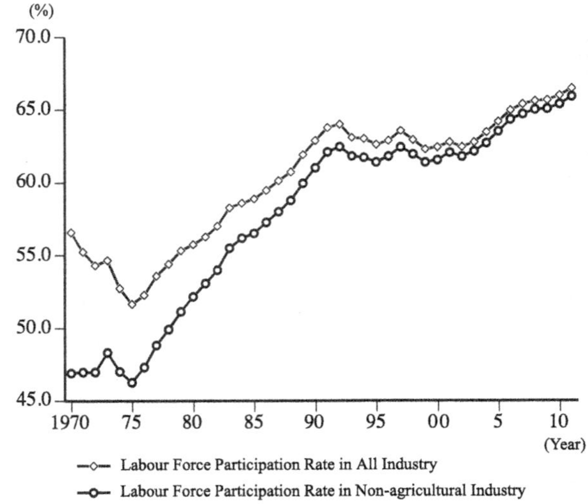

Freiden 1974; Kiernan 1996; Murphy 1987, 1989; Santos 1975; Winegarden 1984). As discussed in Chaps. 1 and 2, these demographic phenomena have mainly been investigated from either an economic or an ideational approach in social sciences. On the other hand, turning to recent social circumstances in Japan, we can easily find factors which affect marriage behaviour in ways that both the economic and ideational approaches predict. In what follows, we will give an overall picture of changing socio-economic circumstances and new developments in people's consciousness in Japan.

The first point to be noted is the clear upward trend of the labour force participation rate for women from the late 1970s onwards (Anderson and Hill 1983; Brinton 1993), although this trend was weakened by the economic recession after the bubble economy burst in the early 1990s. As shown in Graph 3.8, the labour force participant rate of women aged 20–44 stood at around 55 % until 1975 in all industries, but it rose steeply from 55.7 % in 1980 to 65.9 % in 2010. In particular, the tempo of increase for women engaged in non-agricultural industries was remarkably rapid. Indeed, the labour participation rate of women in these industries rose by approximately 13 points from 52.2 % in 1980 to 65.3 % in 2010, whereas it was fluctuating around 50 % until 1980. Because the percentage of female employees in non-agricultural industries is regarded as a proxy for paid employment outside the home, these figures indicate that a growing number of women enjoy many opportunities for paid work outside the home.

Second, the level of education in women has increased remarkably (see Graph 3.9). In 1955, only 5.0 % of women of eligible age went to two-year junior colleges[3] or four-year universities, compared with 15.0 % of men. However, in

[3]The two-year junior college is a type of college offering less strenuous higher education which mainly offers elementary liberal arts and vocational training.

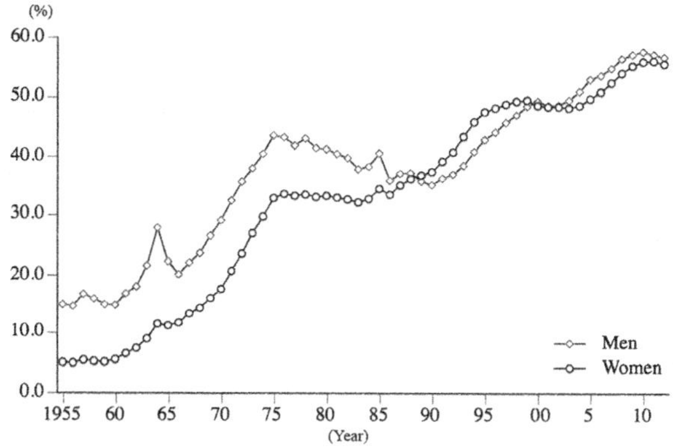

Graph. 3.9 The percentage of men and women going to 2-year colleges and 4-year universities. *Source* The Ministry of Education, Culture, Sports, Science and Technology (various years). School Basic Survey

2012, these figures rose dramatically to 55.6 % for women and 56.6 % for men, respectively, as a result of which the enrolment ratio for women became almost equivalent to the ratio for men. Admittedly, a majority of women went to two-year junior colleges up until the 1970s. Yet, the percentage of students who go onto four-year universities stood at 55.6 % for men and 45.8 % for women in 2012. As a result, the gender gap in the enrolment rate has narrowed considerably. According to the human capital theory (Becker 1975), a rise in educational attainment enhances labour productivity through an investment in human capital. Thus, the rising educational level of women naturally leads to the expansion of female paid employment after university graduation. Indeed, the proportion of university graduates gaining employment (including permanent and contingent work) upon graduation was 70.2 % for women and 58.9 % for men in 2011 (Ministry of Education, Culture, Sports, Science and Technology, Various years). Furthermore, an increase in women's human capital enhances their earning capacity in the labour market, thereby narrowing the gap between men's and women's wages. In fact, the ratio of women's to men's monthly wages in general employees aged 25–29 was only 60.8 % in 1970, while it reached 85.1 % in 2011 (Ministry of Health, Labour and Welfare, Various years).

Based on Becker's economic approach, the above socio-economic changes are undoubtedly driving forces that have discouraged marriage in Japan. More specifically, if women do have very scant employment opportunities and there is a huge wage gap between men and women, the gains from marriage will be large and women's earnings lost on their retreat from the labour market will be small. In such a case, entering into a married status would be a good strategy for maximizing the gains from marriage. In other words, women's specialization in household activities would, in this case, be of higher profit to them. Yet, as women's economic power in the labour market improves and approaches men's power—caused in part by a rise in the female enrolment rate at higher education—single men and women will, from an economic viewpoint, be less willing to marry and trade their surplus. The reason for this is clear: gender specialization in market and domestic work after marriage does not increase women's gains from marriage. Consequently, as women's earning capacity rises, a woman's incentive to marry will diminish. In fact, a multivariate analysis of aggregated prefectural-level data since the 1970s indicates that female hourly wages have a reducing effect on women's marriage probability[4] in Japan (Ogura and Dekle 1992). Similarly, it has been found that Japanese women with high educational credentials tend to remain unmarried more than those with low educational credentials (Raymo 2003a).

It is, however, premature to think that marital behaviour is affected only by economic factors. First, according to the economic theory, if the productivity of men and women was completely equal both in the market sphere and in the domestic sphere, no man and woman would, in theory, marry, since the comparative advantage between both sexes would have disappeared. Yet, it is doubtful whether this is a case in the real world. In fact, the wage gender gap in 2009 was 21.6 in Germany and 12.1 in Denmark (OECD 2011), but the marriage rate in 2009 was 4.6 per 1000 population in the former and 6.0 in the latter. Although the comparative advantage between men's and women's wages is smaller in Denmark than in Germany, the former yields a greater marriage rate than the latter. This evidence suggests that marriage behaviour is not a simple function of earning power (Burgess et al. 2003; Gutiérrez-Domènech 2008).

In the second place, the economic approach does not satisfactorily explain why a considerable number of couples prefer cohabitation to marriage. In 1998, for instance, the proportion of cohabiting women in the 20–24 age group reached 45 % in Denmark, 25 % in France, 39 % in Sweden and 13 % in Britain (Kiernan 1999). Likewise, cohabiting men in the same age group stood at 43, 13, 24 and 12 %, respectively. Cohabiting couples are legally unmarried, but their living arrangements are considerably similar to those of legally married couples. A cohabiting couple lives under one roof, as a married couple does. Thus, there is not a large difference in gains from marriage between married and cohabiting couples. Admittedly, cohabitation, in some cases, ends in marriage, serving as a kind of prelude to marriage (Coleman and Salt 1992). Yet, in other cases, couples continue to cohabit lifelong as an alternative to marriage. Taking these points into consideration, it is difficult to explain the reasons why many adults choose to cohabit only due to economic factors such as wage levels.

Third, women's greater earning capacity may encourage marriage rather than discourage it. For instance, Goldscheider and Waite (1986) find that women's earning power is positively related to their propensity to marry in the USA. This evidence suggests that, even when married life cannot be maintained solely by a man's income, the addition of a woman's income enables the man and woman to marry and make their married life together sustainable (Sweeney 2002). In other words, the economic explanation presumes an asymmetric family where a husband and wife will separately specialize in a single role either in the market or in the home. Yet, due to the double income of a husband and wife, the economic viability of marriage is improved. Hence, as a symmetric family becomes more realistic

[4]Caution is needed when we interpret the statistical result of this study, because it may suffer from the ecological fallacy (see Langbein and Lichtman 1978; Robinson 1950).

and prevailing, women's greater earning capacity may promote their entry into marriage (Oppenheimer 2000; Young and Willmott 1973).

Besides, as discussed in Chap. 2, people's preference for marriage may change in tandem with the development of society one lives in. In other words, it is likely that traditional values are losing support and sway, while individualistic attitudes become stronger than before. In fact, we can see evidence of these trends by pointing to changing attitudes towards marriage among Japanese females. For instance, the several rounds of the Japanese Fertility Survey (National Institute of Population and Social Security Research 2012) shows that more young people have individualistic attitudes. In this survey, unmarried men and women between ages 18 and 34 were asked whether they agree with the opinion that people, after marriage, should have their own purposes in life which differ from their partner's or family's purposes. As shown in Graph 3.10, men and women who agreed that people should have their own purposes in life after marriage gradually increased in percentage, with a particularly conspicuous change occurring in the women surveyed. To be concrete, between the 1992 and the 2010 rounds of this survey, the proportion of respondents supporting the opinion rose from 76.4 to 81.2 % for men and from 78.3 to 84.2 % for women. The percentage of respondents disagreeing with this view, however, fell from 18.2 to 14.9 % for men and from 17.6 to 11.9 % for women. These results suggest that self-oriented attitudes have steadily spread among Japanese people, and a considerable proportion of women no longer seek their happiness only in marriage. It is quite difficult to judge whether this difference of attitude between the surveys was derived from a period effect or

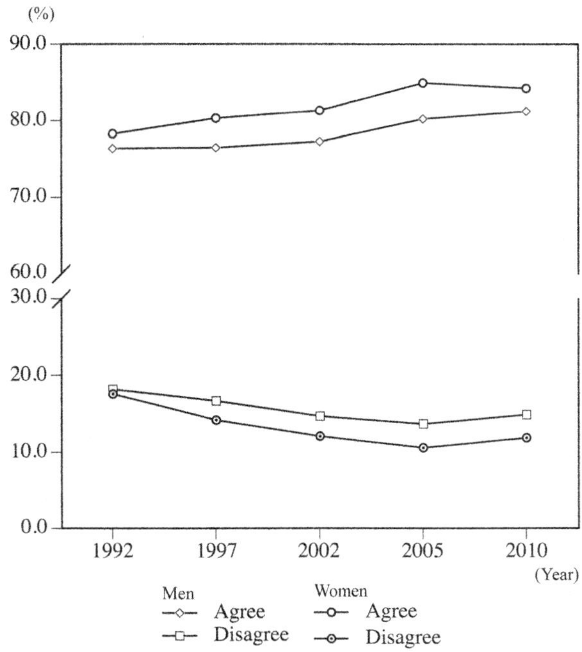

Graph. 3.10 Attitudes to self-oriented lifestyle. *Note* Respondents aged between 18 and 34 were asked the following question: "What do you think about the opinion that people should have their own purposes in life after marriage which are different from their partner's or family's purposes?" *Source* National Institute of Population and Social Security Research (2012). The report on the Fourteenth Japanese National Fertility Survey in 2010

Graph. 3.11 Attitudes towards caring for aged parents. *Source* The Population Problems Research Council of the Mainichi Newspaper (2000). The Japanese population: footsteps of the 50 post-war years

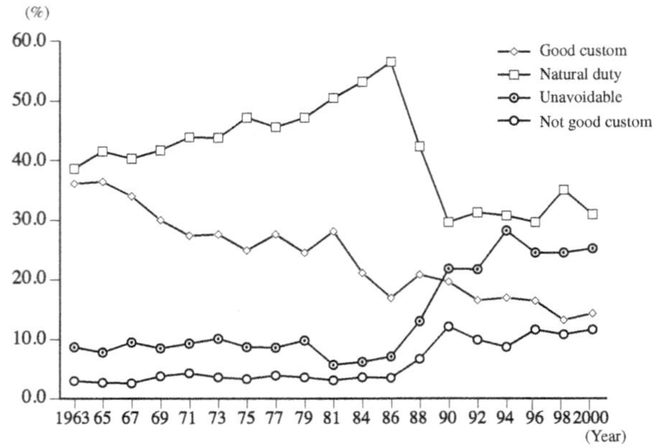

Question: What do you think of children taking care of their aged parents?
Answer:
Good custom: It's a good custom.
Natural duty: It's children's natural duty.
Unavoidable: It's unavoidable, because of a lack of nursing homes or pensins for the aged.
Not good custom: It's not a good custom

a cohort effect (for details, see Chap. 5). In spite of such a drawback, it is safe to say that a substantial number of marriageable adults have a self-oriented attitude towards their lives.

In addition, it seems that conventional values are withering and progressive ideas are spreading in Japan. As is well known, Japanese family relations are influenced by Confucianism, in which great importance has traditionally been attached to the care of aged parents as a filial duty (Dore 1953). Yet, people's attitudes to these traditional inter-generational values appear to have changed. Graph 3.11 displays the trend of attitudes towards caring for aged parents. The proportion of women showing negative attitudes to the care of aged parents increased after the latter half of the 1980s. The percentage of women in the "Unavoidable" category jumped from 5.7 % in 1981 to 25.2 % in 2000. Similarly, the percentage of the "Not good custom" category rose from 3.1 % to 11.6 % during the same period. In contrast, the proportion of women having positive attitudes to the care of aged parents shows a secular downward trend. The percentage of women who thought of caring for aged parents as a good custom reached as much as 38.6 % in 1963, while the figure fell to 14.3 % in 2000. Moreover, the percentage of the "Natural duty" category fell sharply from 56.5 % in 1985 to 30.9 % in 2000 (The Population Problems Research Council of the Mainichi Newspaper 2000). Although we lack definite information on the causes of this drastic fall, it is certain that an increasing number of women have negative attitudes towards the filial obligation.

If people are relying on their children to support them physically and economically in old age, they will be motivated to marry and to have children in order to secure their well-being in their later years[5] (Morgan and Hiroshima 1983;

[5]In a sense, filial obligation can be regarded as a kind of inter-generational wealth-flow mechanism (see Caldwell 1982).

Smith 1981, 1986). In this scenario, young adults choose to delay marriage or to remain celibate could very well jeopardize their well-being in old age. Thus, it becomes a good strategy to have children who will come of age before their retirement. This strategy, however, becomes less attractive when aged people are independent and do not expect assistance and support from their children through a weakening of traditional Confucian values. In short, the motivation to marry and have children may weaken as the level of well-being in old age comes to depend less and less on inter-generational support in a family. Hence, recent marriage patterns in Japan may be attributable to a change in the influence of traditional filial ethics.

As discussed thus far, Japanese socio-economic circumstances and people's attitudes seem to weaken the incentive to marry from a macro-perspective. The rise in women's economic power may reduce their gains from marriage in the way that the economic approach assumes. At the same time, however, people's values and attitudes may discourage marriage and encourage remaining single and pursuing one's own purposes and lifestyle. Thus, we cannot deny that economic and ideational factors affect marriage behaviour in Japan. In the following sections, we will examine the influence of economic and ideational factors on marriage behaviour by using microdata.

3.4 Data and Method for the Analysis of Marriage Behaviour

In the previous section, we discussed economic and attitudinal changes in Japan. With these changes in mind, we cannot deny that Japanese marriage behaviour is influenced by both economic and ideational factors. The primary purpose of this chapter is to examine the effects of economic and ideational factors on marriage behaviour by using our survey data. Yet, before showing the results of the analyses, we will, in this section, describe the data, method and variables used in our analysis.

The present analysis uses data from the Japanese Generations and Gender Survey (JGGS), a nationwide panel survey with a target population of men and women between ages 18 and 69 in Japan. 150,000 individuals were selected by two-stage stratified probability sampling. The first wave of the JGGS was conducted in 2004, and its overall response rate amounted to 57.4 %. The second wave of the survey was carried out in 2007 with 67.5 % of the respondents who answered a questionnaire in the first wave of the survey. The third follow-up survey was conducted in 2010, and its response rate stood at 72.6 % of respondents from the second wave. In this analysis, we selected unmarried men and women at the time of the first survey. As for divorcees, widows and widowers, their remarriage behaviour is likely to be affected by their marital history. However, since the JGGS does not have sufficient information on the marital histories of divorcees, widows and widowers, they were excluded from the present analysis. As a result,

266 men and 358 women between 20 and 45 years of age at the time of the first survey were selected for the analysis.

In the present analysis, we employ the latent class event-history analysis (Hagenaars 1993; Hagenaars and McCutcheon 2002; Vermunt 1997). First of all, we will explain the latent class analysis briefly. Let us suppose that there is one latent (unobserved) variable X with T categories ($t = 1, 2, \ldots T$) and two manifest (observed) variables A with I categories ($i = 1, 2, \ldots I$) and B with J categories ($j = 1, 2, \ldots J$). The model of the latent class analysis is described as follows:

$$\pi_{ijt}^{ABX} = \pi_t^X \pi_{it}^{\bar{A}X} \pi_{jt}^{\bar{B}X}, \quad \text{for } t = 1, 2, \ldots T;\ i = 1, 2, \ldots I;\ j = 1, 2, \ldots J \tag{3.1}$$

where π_{ijt}^{ABX} denotes the probability that an observation which belongs to category i on variable A and to category j on variable B falls in category t on latent variable X. Furthermore, $\pi_{it}^{\bar{A}X}$ denotes the conditional probability that an observation falls in category i on variable A, given that the observation stays at category t on latent variable X. By the same token, $\pi_{jt}^{\bar{B}X}$ denotes the conditional probability that an observation is in category j on variable B, given that the observation stays at category t on latent variable X. Here, a great probability of $\pi_{it}^{\bar{A}X}$ means that category i on variable A has a strong connection to category t on latent variable X. In contrast, a small probability of $\pi_{it}^{\bar{A}X}$ means that category i on variable A has a weak connection to category t on latent variable X. In short, the latent class analysis finds out some latent categories based on the response patterns of observed variables.

The latent class event-history analysis is a hazard analysis including manifest and latent variables as covariates. The model of the analysis is expressed as follows:

$$h(t) = \frac{\exp\left(\alpha + \gamma_k w_k + \sum \beta_j x_j\right)}{1 + \exp\left(\alpha + \gamma_k w_k + \sum \beta_j x_j\right)} \tag{3.2}$$

Here, $h(t)$ is the probability of occurring an event at time t; α is a constant term; w_k is a category k of latent variable w; γ_k is a parameter of the category; x_j is a manifest independent variable x; and β_j is a parameter of the variable.

$$\log\left[\frac{h(t)}{1 - h(t)}\right] = \alpha + \gamma_k w_k + \sum \beta_j x_j \tag{3.3}$$

After taking the logit transformation of (3.2), Eq. (3.3) indicates the discrete-time hazard model. The important feature of this model is that it distinguishes between the effects of both manifest and latent covariates on event occurrences. In this analysis, we examine the probability of getting married after the first wave of the JGGS. The dependent variable is, therefore, the hazard rate of respondents experiencing their first marriage after the year 2004.

A noteworthy point is that the panel data of the JGGS suffer sample attrition. As mentioned before, since the response rate of the second wave of the survey stood at 67.5, 32.5 % of respondents who answered the first-survey questionnaire dropped out of our samples. Similarly, due to sample attrition, the number of respondents was reduced by 27.4 % from the second wave to the third wave of the survey. If only the remaining samples are analysed, estimated parameters may be distorted by sample attrition. Taking this point into consideration, we use propensity score weighting in order to exclude a bias caused by sample attrition (Guo and Fraser 2014). More specifically, the probability of a respondent's remaining in the sample was first estimated by logistic regression.[6] Then, an inverse of the estimated probability is used as a value of sample weight. As for independent variables, we use the following variable in the analysis.

3.4.1 Socio-economic Variables

In the present analysis, the effects of two socio-economic variables on marriage will be examined. The first variable is the level of income. According to the economic approach to marriage behaviour, women with high earning power in the labour market have less to gain from marriage than women with low earning power. As a result, the increase in women's income weakens the advantages once held by women who specialized in household activities after marriage. This may attenuate women's incentive to marry. At the same time, it is, however, possible that women's higher income encourages marriage. As discussed previously, if a woman's high income serves to improve the economic viability of marriage and enhance well-being in married life, high-salaried women are more likely to marry than low-salaried women. Hence, we cannot hypothesize the effect of women's income a priori. As for men's income, it is expected that their greater earning power contributes to stabilizing and sustaining family life after marriage (Kalmijn 2011; Oppenheimer 1998, 2000). Thus, adult men with a high income are more likely to marry than those with a low income. In this analysis, the respondent's annual income was divided into four categories: (1) less than 2,000,000 yen; (2) 2,000,000–2,990,000 yen; (3) 3,000,000–3,990,000 yen; and (4) equal or more than 4,000,000 yen.

The second variable is occupation. As is the case with income, we can expect two different relations between women's occupation and their marriage behaviour. One of these relations is a negative effect that women's occupation places on

[6]The propensity scores were calculated by the following logistic regression.

$$\begin{aligned}\log\left(\frac{q}{1-q}\right) &= \alpha + \beta_1(\text{sex}) + \beta_2(\text{age}) + \beta_3(\text{marital status}) \\ &\quad + \beta_4(\text{the years of living in your current house}) \\ &\quad + \beta_5(\text{educational attainment}) + \beta_6(\text{residential prefecture}) \\ &\quad + \beta_7(\text{the number of children ever-born})\end{aligned}$$

Here, q is the probability of respondents remaining in our sample.

marriage, as expected from Becker's economic theory, which assumes that a key factor in marriage decision-making lies in gains from marriage. As previously discussed, a woman whose economic power is equal to that of her partner will have only small prospective gains from marriage. Hence, it is expected that, owing to the diminution of gains from marriage, women working in high-salary occupations such as professional and managerial jobs will be less willing to trade surpluses with men than those working in low-salary occupations such as manual jobs. This will consequently make women in high-salary occupations more reluctant to marry, leading to a delay or an avoidance of marriage. It should be, however, borne in mind that this hypothesis appears to be irrelevant to people engaged in agriculture and to those who are self-employed. Becker's theory implicitly presumes that, after marriage, one devotes oneself either to housework or to work outside the home. Yet, productive work is, to some extent, compatible with housework for women engaged in agriculture and those who are self-employed, since their home and workplace are usually the same or adjacent to each other. In such working conditions, even if a woman has a high earning capacity, she can continue to work after marriage. In this case, prospective gains from marriage will have little effect on deciding whether to marry.

The above hypothesis posits a negative relation between women's occupation and marriage. At the same time, however, good employment opportunities for women, such as professional and managerial occupations, may encourage marriage (Goode 1963). It is possible that a great female earning power can enhance the viability of a new household after marriage (Piotrowski et al. 2015). In fact, it is found that where "neo-localism" is a strong rule of household formation, a rise in the economic stability of a new household brought about by a wife's employment has a positive relation to nuptiality (Hajnal 1965, 1983; Schofield 1989). Hence, women working in high-salaried occupations such as professional or managerial jobs may marry early and be unlikely to remain single.

The effect of men's occupation on their marriage behaviour is expected to be similar to that of men's wages. As is the case with wages, good employment opportunities for men bring higher earning power and serve to enhance the viability and sustainability of married life. With this point in mind, we hypothesize that adult men working in a high-salaried occupation are more likely to marry than those working in a low-salaried occupation. In the present analysis, we classified the respondent's occupation into four categories: (1) out of employment; (2) professional and managerial; (3) clerical, sales and service; and (3) manual, agriculture, fishery and others.

3.4.2 Ideational and Attitudinal Variables

As discussed in Sect. 3.2, the ideational theory claims that the attenuation of traditional values and the strengthening of self-oriented consciousness affect the patterns of family formation in Western countries (Ariès 1980; Lesthaeghe 1983, 1995;

Lesthaeghe and Meekers 1986; Lesthaeghe and Surkyn 1988; Simons 1986a, b; van de Kaa 1987). Since the JGGS included questions on respondents' attitude towards marriage and family, it was used to examine the effects of ideational factors on marriage behaviour. In concrete terms, we used the following six opinion items for our analysis:

1. The main purpose of marriage is to have children.
2. It is all right for a man and woman to live together without being married.
3. It is much better for everyone if the man earns the main living and the woman takes care of the home and family.
4. Parents should provide financial help for their adult children when the children are having financial difficulties.
5. A man can have a full and satisfying life without marrying (only for men).
6. A woman can have a full and satisfying life without marrying (only for women).

Five answering categories were provided for each statement in the questionnaire: (1) Strongly agree, (2) Agree, (3) Uncertain, (4) Disagree and (5) Strongly disagree. For each opinion item, respondents were asked to choose the single answering category closest to their view at the time of the survey. For the sake of convenience, if a respondent chose "Strongly agree" or "Agree", we combined them into the "Agree" group in this analysis. Likewise, if a respondent chose "Disagree" or "Strongly disagree", they were placed in the "Disagree" category. We will examine the influence of attitudes on marriage behaviour by using these categorical variables.

3.4.3 Family-Related Variables

Three variables relating to family and life course are used in this analysis. The first variable is co-residence with parents. It should be pointed out that, in Mediterranean countries, the delay in marriage is strongly linked to the longer residence of young adults in the parental home (Billari and Rosina 2004). In these countries, due to a strong emotional tie between parents and children, people tend to equate their own well-being with their family's well-being (Reher 2004). As a result, parents make their home a materially and psychologically comfortable place for their children, thereby weakening any incentive to leave the parental home and to marry (Zuanna 2004). In fact, age at leaving the parental home is later in Southern Europe than in North-western Europe (Iacovou and Parisi 2009). For example, median age at leaving the parental home was 21.4 for men and 20.3 for women in Denmark in 1994, while the figures rose up to age 29.7 and age 27.1, respectively, in Italy. A similar strong tie between parents and children is also observed in Japan (Zuanna et al. 1998). Bearing this in mind, we expect that co-residence with parents will reduce the risk of marriage.

The second variable is a respondent's birth order. If a family line is maintained by primogeniture, the first-born child will suffer from stronger social pressure to marry than a second or a third child. In such a family system, it is a desirable strategy for the first-born child to marry as early as possible and have a child to succeed in the family line. A second or third child, however, will be free from this duty. Hence, a second or third child will remain single or marry later than a first-born child. In particular, because Japanese society has held the cultural tradition of the patrilineal family system, or the so-called '*Ie*', parental pressure to marry is most likely to be put on the first-born son. Daughters also may be free from the familial pressure to marriage. Yet, it is possible that a first-born daughter without any male siblings is strongly urged to marry early, because she must serve in the place of a male heir for the continuation of her family line.

The effect of this variable on marriage is, however, unclear in contemporary Japan. If maintaining a family line is no longer a principal concern in Japanese society, this variable will not affect marriage behaviour. For instance, the proportion of people who thought that continuing the family line was important fell remarkably from 74.0 % in 1953 to 21.0 % in 2008, whereas the percentage of respondents who did not place special value on the continuance of a family line rose steeply from 16.0 to 57.0 % in the same period (The Institute of Statistical Mathematics 2009). Thus, the effect of this variable cannot be determined a priori.

The third variable is the experience of cohabitation before marriage. As mentioned before, the proportion of Japanese young adults who experience cohabitation is on the increase. Generally speaking, cohabitation can be classified into two types. The first type of cohabitation is a prelude to legal marriage, where the couple will in most cases end up entering into a legal marriage. The second type of cohabitation is an alternative to legal marriage, where the couple will remain legally unmarried for a long period. If the first type of cohabitation increases in number, the risk of marriage will be greater for young adults who have ever cohabited than those who never cohabited. In Japan, 58 % of cohabiting unions resulted in marriage in 2004 (Raymo et al. 2009), which indicates that the first type of cohabitation slightly outnumbers the second type. Hence, it is expected that the experience of cohabitation enhances the risk of marriage in Japan.

3.4.4 Control Variables

Three demographic variables are employed as control variables. The first variable is the respondents' birth cohorts. Popular wisdom has it that one's birth cohort plays an important role in shaping one's life course (Giele and Elder 1998; Mortimer and Shanahan 2003; Ryder 1965); it is assumed that people born in the same cohort share a similar experience, which affects their life perspective or life purpose. For instance, it is pointed out that children who experienced the great depression in adolescence tended to be independent earlier (Elder 1977). It is therefore likely that respondents' birth cohorts affect their marriage behaviour. In this analysis, we included four birth cohorts in our model: (1) before 1969; (2) 1970–1974; (3) 1975–1979; and (4) after 1980.

The second variable is a respondent's age. As is well known, the risk of entering into married status is affected by age. For example, the lower age limit is regulated by law. In addition, since the age of school entrance and graduation is prescribed, the risk of marriage is also affected by age as far as student marriage occurs scarcely. Based on the results of our preliminary analysis, we will divide respondents' age into four groups: (1) under 24; (2) 25–29; (3) 30–34; and (4) over 35. The present analysis will use these respondents' ages as a control variable.

The third variable is premarital pregnancy. As shown in Graph 3.6, the percentage of pregnancy-dependent marriage is on the rise in Japan. If the entry into married status is strongly affected by a premarital conception, the influence of economic and ideational factors on marriage behaviour will not be examined precisely. Thus, in order to examine the net effect of these factors, we need to partial out the influence of premarital pregnancy. In the present analysis, we define premarital pregnancy as the case where a child was born to a couple within eight months of their marriage and control its influence on marriage behaviour.

3.5 Descriptive Analysis of Marriage Patterns

The primary purpose of this analysis is to examine marriage behaviour by applying latent class event-history analysis to our survey data. Before showing the results of the analysis, we will, in this section, provide an overall picture of marriage patterns by using the survey data. In particular, we will focus on exploring the relation between marriage behaviour and the variables presented in the previous section.

Table 3.1 displays the percentage of respondents who got married by the third wave of the survey, according to respondents' income levels. Overall, a higher male income tends to yield a higher percentage of marriage. For instance, 24.4 % of men

Table 3.1 Annual income and marriage (%)

	Marital status		
	Single	Married	*N*
Men's income (at wave 1)			
Less than 2,000,000 yen	89.6	10.4	115
2,000,000–2,990,000 yen	81.4	18.6	59
3,000,000–3,990,000 yen	63.8	36.2	47
4,000,000 yen–	75.6	24.4	45
N	215	51	266
Women's income (at wave 1)			
Less than 2,000,000 yen	85.4	14.6	226
2,000,000–2,990,000 yen	69.0	31.0	71
3,000,000–3,990,000 yen	69.7	30.3	33
4,000,000 yen–	82.1	17.9	28
N	288	70	358

Source The Japanese Generations and Gender Survey

who earned greater than or equal to 4,000,000 yen a year entered into marriage by the third wave of the survey, while only 10.4 % of those who earned less than 2,000,000 yen got married in the same period. Similarly, the percentage is relatively low for men even in the "2,000,000–2,990,000 yen" category. Unlike the case of men, the results for women do not show a clear linear relation between income and marriage. Admittedly, the lowest percentage, 14.6 %, was observed in women in the smallest income group. Yet, the second lowest percentage rested with the highest income group. In fact, only 17.9 % of women in this highest income category entered into marriage over the course of six years. By contrast, women in the mid-range income groups showed a higher marriage percentage. The percentage of women who got married by the third wave of the survey reached 31.0 % in the "2,000,000–2,990,000 yen" category and 30.3 % in the "3,000,000–3,990,000 yen" category. According to the new home economic theory, the high earning power of a woman should reduce a probability of marriage by a decrease in the gains from marriage. Yet, the percentage of married women does not decrease as their income rises. On the other hand, if a great earning increases the economic viability of marriage and enhances well-being in married life, the percentage of married adults should increase in tandem with a rise in their income. Such a consistent relation, however, is not clearly identified in Table 3.1. Hence, as far as Table 3.1 shows, the relation between income and marriage behaviour is not perfectly fitted to the economic explanations.

Concerning a respondent's occupation, the "professional" and the "clerical" category showed a large percentage of married men, while the "out of employment" and the "manual" category had a small percentage (see Table 3.2). To take an example, the percentage of married men reached 25.9 % in the "professional" group, while that figure fell to only 5.7 % in the "out of employment" group. Likewise, 30.2 % of women in a professional or a managerial job got married, whereas only 12.1 % of unemployed women entered into marriage. Due to their

Table 3.2 Occupation and marriage (%)

	Marital status		
	Single	Married	*N*
Men's occupation (at wave 1)			
Out of employment	94.3	5.7	70
Professional/managerial	74.1	25.9	27
Clerical/sales/service	73.0	27.0	74
Manual/agriculture/other	79.0	21.1	95
N	215	51	266
Women's occupation (at wave 1)			
Out of employment	87.9	12.1	99
Professional/managerial	69.8	30.2	43
Clerical/sales/service	76.7	23.3	189
Manual/agriculture/other	96.3	3.7	27
N	288	70	358

Source The Japanese Generations and Gender Survey

Table 3.3 Co-residence and marriage (%)

	Marital status		
	Single	Married	*N*
Men's living arrangements (at wave 1)			
Living with parents	83.2	16.8	232
Not living with parents	64.7	35.3	34
N	215	51	266
Women's living arrangements (at wave 1)			
Living with parents	82.7	17.3	52
Not living with parents	80.1	19.9	306
N	288	70	358

Source The Japanese Generations and Gender Survey

high income and stable employment, people working in a professional or managerial occupation should have a more enhanced viability of marriage, compared with those who are out of employment or engaged in a manual job. This disparity may lead to a different probability of marriage in Table 3.2. Thus, we may argue that upper social classes enjoy a greater chance of getting married than lower classes.

Next, we shall turn to variables relating to family and life course. Table 3.3 displays the relation between parental co-residence and marriage. Interestingly, co-residence with parents impacts on sons in considerably different ways from daughters where their marriage percentages are concerned. More specifically, when sons lived with their parents, only 16.8 % of them married by the third wave of the survey. Yet, when sons lived independently of their parents, fully 35.3 % of them got married. This evidence indicates that co-residence with parents inhibits male marriage. In contrast, such an inhibitive effect is not identified for women. Indeed, 17.3 % of daughters who lived with their parents entered into marriage, while 19.9 % of daughters who did not live with their parents married by the third survey. It therefore follows that co-residence with parents brings no difference in daughters' marriage probability.

A similar relation was observed with regard to birth order (see Table 3.4). Male and female birth orders display quite different marriage patterns. To be specific, 21.4 % of first sons entered into marriage, whereas the percentage stayed at only 17.0 % for not-first sons. In short, the probability of marriage is greater for first than not-first sons. By contrast, such a difference was not clearly found among daughters. The proportion of married women was 19.1 % for first daughters, while this figure stood at 20.3 % for not-first daughters. As far as this evidence shows, there is no salient difference in marriage probability between first and not-first daughters.

Likewise, the experience of cohabitation appears to impact in striking contrast on men's and women's marriage patterns (see Table 3.5). Fully 42.9 % of men who had ever experienced cohabitation eventually married. Meanwhile, the percentage of married men with no experience of cohabitation was only 16.4 %. It, therefore, follows that cohabitation experience encourages men to marriage. In contrast,

Table 3.4 Birth order and marriage (%)

	Marital status		
	Single	Married	*N*
Men's birth order (at wave 1)			
First son	78.6	21.4	131
Other sons	83.0	17.0	135
N	215	51	266
Women's birth order (at wave 1)			
First daughter	81.0	19.1	210
Other daughters	79.7	20.3	148
N	288	70	358

Source The Japanese Generations and Gender Survey

Table 3.5 Cohabitation experience and marriage (%)

	Marital status		
	Single	Married	*N*
Men's cohabitation (at wave 1)			
Ever-cohabited	57.1	42.9	28
Never-cohabited	83.6	16.4	238
N	215	51	266
Women's cohabitation (at wave 1)			
Ever-cohabited	77.4	22.6	31
Never-cohabited	80.7	19.3	327
N	288	70	358

Source The Japanese Generations and Gender Survey

cohabitation does not have a conspicuous impact on female marriage behaviour. In fact, 22.6 % of women who experienced cohabitation married, while 19.3 % of those who never cohabited also got married. It follows that the risk of marriage in ever-cohabited and never-cohabited women does not substantially differ.

Finally, we will look at the relation between marriage and ideational factors. Table 3.6 shows marital status by displaying six opinion items that measure respondents' attitudes. As for men, conservative attitudes and a strong commitment to traditional values appear to lead a higher probability of marriage. For instance, 20.6 % of men who supported traditional gender roles (Item C) got married, while 18.3 % of men who did not subscribe to traditional gender roles entered into marriage. Similarly, in Item D, the percentage of married men reached 24.1 % for those who supported traditional values on inter-generational relationships, whereas the figure fell to 18.0 % among those who disagreed with these values. Moreover, 20.4 % of men who disagreed with cohabitation (Item B) married, while 17.4 % of men who agreed with cohabitation entered into marriage. As for women, a clear relation was not identified between attitudes and marital status. For instance, the percentage of married women reached 16.7 % for those who disagree with cohabitation (Item B), whereas the figure slightly rose up to 18.0 % for women who agree with it. Likewise, 19.2 % of women who agreed with

Table 3.6 Value-orientations and marriage (%)

Men (at wave 1)	Marital status			Women (at wave 1)	Marital status		
	Single	Married	*N*		Single	Married	*N*
(a) The main purpose of marriage is to have children							
Agree	83.0	17.0	53	Agree	82.7	17.3	52
Uncertain	81.6	18.4	147	Uncertain	82.1	17.9	151
Disagree	77.3	22.7	66	Disagree	78.1	21.9	155
N	215	51	266	N	288	70	358
(b) It is all right for a man and woman to live together without being married							
Agree	82.6	17.4	132	Agree	82.0	18.0	217
Uncertain	78.8	21.3	80	Uncertain	75.3	24.7	93
Disagree	79.6	20.4	54	Disagree	83.3	16.7	48
N	215	51	266	*N*	288	70	358
(c) It is much better for everyone if the man earns the main living and the woman takes care of the home and family							
Agree	79.5	20.6	73	Agree	83.6	16.4	67
Uncertain	81.2	18.8	133	Uncertain	80.4	19.6	153
Disagree	81.7	18.3	60	Disagree	79.0	21.0	138
N	215	51	266	*N*	288	70	358
(d) Parents should provide financial help for their adult children when the children are having financial difficulties							
Agree	75.9	24.1	83	Agree	80.9	19.2	94
Uncertain	83.5	16.5	133	Uncertain	79.9	20.1	189
Disagree	82.0	18.0	50	Disagree	81.3	18.7	75
N	215	51	266	*N*	288	70	358
(e) A man can have a full and satisfying life without marrying				*(f) A woman can have a full and satisfying life without marrying*			
Agree	85.9	14.1	85	Agree	87.9	12.1	141
Uncertain	82.9	17.1	140	Uncertain	76.0	24.0	154
Disagree	63.4	36.6	41	Disagree	74.6	25.4	63
N	215	51	266	*N*	288	70	358

Source The Japanese Generations and Gender Survey

inter-generational financial support (Item D) got married, while the figure stood at 18.7 % of those women who disagreed with this opinion item. Interestingly, the proportion of married people was greatest for both men and women who disagreed that the main purpose of marriage is to have children (Item A). This evidence implies that people who psychologically disconnect human procreation from marriage have a greater risk of marriage, regardless of their sex.

We cannot, of course, draw a definite conclusion from this descriptive analysis of marriage patterns, for it does not partial out the confounding effect of variables. Thus, we will, in the following sections, carry out latent class event-history analysis to examine the net effect of these variables.

3.6 Finding Latent Classes for Marriage Behaviour

In the latter part of the previous section, we showed the relation between attitudinal factors and marriage behaviour. Yet, since respondents' attitudes are measured by multiple items, it is quite difficult to understand the overall relation between attitudes and marriage behaviour. Taking this point into consideration, we will, in this section, classify respondents' attitudes into a few groups by using latent class analysis.

Table 3.7 displays the model evaluation of latent class analysis. As for men, the chi-square test is statistically significant for the 2-class model, indicating that the model is quite different from an unconstrained model. Thus, two latent classes are not appropriate for classifying respondents' attitudes. However, since the 3-class and 4-class models were insignificant in the chi-square test at the 10 % level, they do not differ from the null model and have a sufficient goodness of fit to divide respondents' attitudes. Yet, the value of Bayesian information criterion (BIC) is smaller for the 3-class model than for the 4-class model. Since a smaller BIC's value means a better fit of a model (Raftery 1995), we can argue that the 3-class model is most appropriate for a classification of men's attitudes. With regard to women, the classification of attitudes is similar to that of men. The chi-square test is significant for the female 2-class model, thereby making it considerably different from the null model. We can, hence, conclude that the 2-class model is not appropriate for classifying respondents' attitudes. In contrast, the 3-class and 4-class models were insignificant at 10 % level with the chi-square test, so that both models are not different from an unconstrained model. Yet, the value of BIC is smaller for the 3-class model than for the 4-class model. Thus, we can conclude that the 3-class model is most fitted to distinguishing women's attitudes.

Now, let us turn to an interpretation of the 3-latent classes model. Table 3.8 shows the relation between the latent classes and the conditional probability of each opinion item. As for men's latent classes, Class 1 yields a relatively high probability in the "Agree" category of Items (3), (4) and (5). For example, the probability of agreeing that it is much better for everyone if the man earns the

Table 3.7 Model evaluation of latent class analysis

Number of latent classes	Degrees of freedom	Log likelihood	Chi-square *p*-value	BIC	*N*
Husbands					
2	221	−1328.22	0.01	2773.70	266
3	210	−1310.92	0.23	2800.52	266
4	199	−1296.83	0.50	2833.76	266
Wives					
2	221	−1771.65	0.01	3666.78	358
3	210	−1743.98	0.39	3676.14	358
4	199	−1735.17	0.55	3723.21	358

Source The Japanese Generations and Gender Survey

Table 3.8 Latent class and conditional probability

Men				Women			
	Class 1	Class 2	Class 3		Class 1	Class 2	Class 3
Item (1)				Item (1)			
Agree	0.31	0.09	0.19	Agree	0.34	0.11	0.04
Uncertain	0.63	0.62	0.23	Uncertain	0.37	0.72	0.15
Disagree	0.06	0.30	0.59	Disagree	0.29	0.17	0.81
Item (2)				Item (2)			
Agree	0.46	0.42	0.81	Agree	0.46	0.57	0.75
Uncertain	0.06	0.47	0.18	Uncertain	0.18	0.41	0.17
Disagree	0.48	0.11	0.01	Disagree	0.36	0.02	0.08
Item (3)				Item (3)			
Agree	0.60	0.07	0.19	Agree	0.55	0.11	0.01
Uncertain	0.29	0.81	0.02	Uncertain	0.35	0.62	0.29
Disagree	0.11	0.12	0.79	Disagree	0.11	0.27	0.71
Item (4)				Items (4)			
Agree	0.44	0.27	0.07	Agree	0.36	0.23	0.23
Uncertain	0.29	0.68	0.42	Uncertain	0.43	0.63	0.50
Disagree	0.27	0.05	0.50	Disagree	0.22	0.14	0.27
Item (5)				Item (6)			
Agree	0.37	0.28	0.32	Agree	0.32	0.30	0.55
Uncertain	0.47	0.64	0.36	Uncertain	0.27	0.70	0.26
Disagree	0.16	0.08	0.32	Disagree	0.41	0.00	0.18
Overall class size	0.34	0.51	0.15	Overall class size	0.27	0.37	0.36

Item statements are as follows:
(1) The main purpose of marriage is to have children
(2) It is all right for a man and woman to live together without being married
(3) It is much better for everyone if the man earns the main living and the woman takes care of the home and family
(4) Parents should provide financial help for their adult children when the children are having financial difficulties
(5) A man can have a full and satisfying life without marrying (only for men)
(6) A woman can have a full and satisfying life without marrying (only for women)
Source The Japanese Generations and Gender Survey

main living and the woman takes care of the home and family (Item 3) reached 0.60. In addition, the conditional probability of the "Agree" category in Item (4) stood at 0.44, while that of the "Disagree" category was 0.27. Since Items (3), (4) and (5) indicate the level of accepting traditional values, it follows that respondents who agree with these statements display a conservative attitude. Thus, Class 1 can be termed a "conservative" group. With regard to Class 2, its most conspicuous feature is the fact that the "Uncertain" category displays a higher probability in all items. For instance, the probability of the "Uncertain" category was 0.81 for Item (3), 0.68 for Item (4) and 0.64 for Item (5). This response pattern indicates that respondents in this group do not show a decisive view about the opinion items. Class 2 can therefore be named a "neutral" group. Class 3 yields a high probability in the "Disagree" category in Items (1), (3) and (4). To take an example, the probability for disagreeing with the idea that it is much better for everyone if the man earns the main living and the woman takes care of the home and family (Item 3) fully reached 0.79. By contrast, the probability for agreeing that it is all right for a man and woman to live together without being married (Item 2) stood at 0.81 in Class 3. Since disagreeing with Items (1), (3) and (4) and agreeing with Item (2) mean that respondents are in opposition to conventional values, this class can therefore be called a "progressive" group.

With regard to women, Class 1 shows a great probability in the "Agree" category of Item (3). More specifically, the probability for agreeing that it is much better for everyone if the man earns the main living and the woman takes care of the home and family (Item 3) reached 0.55. Furthermore, compared with the other two latent classes, Class 1 showed a relatively large probability in the "Disagree" category in Items (2) and (6). Since agreeing with Item (3) and disagreeing with Items (2) and (6) can be regarded as an indication of support for traditional values, Class 1 can therefore be termed a "conservative" group. In Class 2, many women tended to choose the "Uncertain" category. The probability for falling into this category reached 0.72 in Item (1) and 0.70 in Item (6). Even in the remaining items, the "Uncertain" category yields a relatively high value. Judging from this response pattern, Class 2 can be classified as a "neutral" group. In contrast to Class 1, Class 3 has a response pattern expressing opposition to conventional values on marriage and family. For instance, the probability for disagreeing with the idea that the main purpose of marriage is to have children (Item 1) reached 0.81 in Class 3. Likewise, women in Class 3 belong to the "Agree" category of Item (2) with a probability of 0.75. These response patterns indicate that women in Class 3 are in opposition to traditional ideas on marriage and family relation. As far as these patterns show, then, we may call this class a "progressive" group.

What is interesting is that there is a gender difference in the overall size of the three latent classes. The conservative group is considerably large for men, commanding 34 % of all men, whereas the progress group is smallest and composed of only 15 %. In contrast, the progressive category is the second largest latent class, containing 36 % of the female respondents, although the conservative category stood at no more than 27 %. Thus, we can argue that Japanese men are more conservative than Japanese women in terms of their attitudes towards marriage and family.

3.7 Results of the Latent Class Event-History Analysis of Marriage

The results of our latent class event-history analysis for male marriage are displayed in Table 3.9. The first impression of Model 1 in Table 3.9 is that men's income plays an important role in marriage behaviour. To be specific, as men's

Table 3.9 Results of latent class event-history analysis for men

	Model 1	Model 2	Model 3	Model 4	Model 5	Model 6
Covariate	Coefficient	Coefficient	Coefficient	Coefficient	Coefficient	Coefficient
Constant	−1.91**	−1.77*	−2.48***	−3.68***	−2.24**	−1.60**
Men's age+						
Under 24	2.22**	1.26*	2.43**	2.48**	1.54**	2.09**
25–29	1.34**	0.98**	1.31**	1.32**	1.41**	1.29**
(30–34)						
Over 35	−0.04	−0.02	−0.18	−0.32	−0.60	−0.20
Birth cohort						
Before 1969	−1.20	−1.29	−0.94	−0.46	−1.71	−0.58
1970–1974	0.26	0.01	0.24	0.30	0.67	0.31
(1975–1979)						
After 1980	−1.37*	−1.27*	−1.39**	−1.50**	−0.61*	−1.24*
Birth order						
First son	0.30	0.28	0.25	0.30		
(Other)						
Co-residence with parents+						
Yes	−1.86***	−1.83***			−2.25**	−1.89***
(No)						
Men's income+						
(Less than 2,000,000 yen)						
2,000,000–2,990,000 yen	0.69		0.67	0.65	1.32	0.67
3,000,000–3,990,000 yen	1.76***		1.77***	1.68***	2.66*	1.85***
4,000,000 yen	1.86***		1.87***	1.67***	2.99*	2.05***
Men's occupation+						
(Out of employment)						
Professional/managerial		1.57**				
Clerical/sales/service		1.52**				
Manual/agriculture/other		1.37**				
Cohabitation experience before marriage+						
Yes			0.78**	0.63		
(No)						
Premarital pregnancy+						
Yes	1.28**	1.58**		1.15*		
(No)						
Latent class						

(continued)

Table 3.9 (continued)

	Model 1	Model 2	Model 3	Model 4	Model 5	Model 6
Covariate	Coefficient	Coefficient	Coefficient	Coefficient	Coefficient	Coefficient
(Neutral)						
Conservative					2.12*	
Progressive					−1.04	
Log likelihood	−493.49	−511.74	−638.66	−645.84	-602.48	−665.32
BIC	157.81	194.31	159.46	156.25	145.58	146.68
N	266	266	266	266	266	266

Reference categories in parentheses
+ is a time-varying covariate
Time-varying variables take values prior to the occurrence of an event
$*p < 0.10$; $**p < 0.05$; $***p < 0.01$
Source The Japanese Generations and Gender Survey

income increases, more men enter into marriage. For instance, the risk of getting married is 6.5 times greater for men earning 3,000,000–3,990,000 yen a year than for those earning less than less than 2,000,000 yen. Furthermore, when men's annual income amounted to greater than or equal to 4,000,000 yen, the risk of their marrying was 7.9 times greater than the risk of men earning the least income. These findings indicate that, due to the strong economic viability and stability of livelihood, men with a higher earning capacity enter into marriage more frequently.

As for co-residence with parents, fewer men who lived with their parents married than men who did not live with their parents. The hazard rate for men living with parents was 85 % lower than the rate for men not living with parents. As mentioned earlier in this chapter, the long duration of residence among young adults in the parental home is connected to the delay in marriage in Mediterranean countries (Billari and Rosina 2004). As is the case in these countries, due to a strong parent–child attachment, co-residence with parents may provide sons with comfortable living arrangements in Japan. Indeed, since domestic work such as washing, cooking and cleaning is mainly performed by mothers, living in the parental home is quite convenient for unmarried sons. As a result of this, it is likely that co-residence with parents significantly reduces the hazard rate of male marriage.

Interestingly, the birth order of sons did not show a statistically significant effect on the hazard rate of marriage. The "*Ie*" family system is often referred to as the Japanese cultural tradition of primogeniture. If this system remains influential to the family formation process, the first son should marry earlier than other sons in order to maintain his family line successfully. Yet, the results of our analysis reveal that there is no difference in the risk of marriage of first sons and other sons. Thus, we may argue that the influence of the "*Ie*" family system is very weak in contemporary Japan.

With regard to men's occupations, the "professional" category revealed the greatest and significant coefficient (see Table 3.9, Model 2). In concrete terms, men engaged in a professional or a managerial job had a 5.2 times greater hazard rate of marriage than those who were out of employment. Similarly, the "clerical" group and the "manual" group also yielded a statistically significant coefficient. The hazard rates for both groups were approximately 4.9 times greater than the rates for the "out of employment" group. This evidence suggests that economic stability plays a crucial role in determining whether men marry. To put it another way, men who remain out of employment can rarely enter into marriage, due to a lack of economic resources.

Models 3 and 4 of Table 3.9 were prepared to examine the effects of cohabitation on marriage behaviour. As might be expected, the experience of cohabitation increases the risk of marriage significantly (see Table 3.9, Model 3). The hazard rate of marriage was 2.2 times greater for men who had experienced cohabitation than for men who had never experienced it. Yet, the cohabitation variable becomes insignificant in Model 4 of Table 3.9 after we control the influence of premarital pregnancy on entry into marriage. The coefficient of premarital pregnancy is, nevertheless, statistically significant. The risk of marriage was 3.2 times greater for men with a premarital pregnancy than for men without a premarital pregnancy. In short, when controlling for the effect of premarital pregnancy, cohabitation does not increase the risk of marriage. In other words, it may be that the probability of marriage increases in magnitude not through cohabitation itself, but through premarital conception and pregnancy resulting from cohabitation.

In terms of ideational factors, men with conservative attitudes significantly increase a risk of marriage (see Table 3.9, Model 5). Compared to men with neutral attitudes, men with conservative attitudes yielded an 8.3 times greater risk of marriage. We can, therefore, argue that not only economic but also ideational factors affect male marriage behaviour. It should, however, be borne in mind that the influence of ideational factors is not so strong. According to the result of the log-likelihood ratio test, Model 5 of Table 3.9 is more fitted than Model 6 excluding the attitudinal variables from Model 5. Yet, the value of BIC is slightly smaller in Model 5 of Table 3.9 than in Model 6 of the same table. Thus, judging from this value, there is only a very small difference in the goodness of fit between the model with ideational variables and the model without them.

Now let us turn to women's marriage. Table 3.10 displays the results of women's latent class event-history analysis. As is the case of men, high-salaried women had a significantly higher hazard rate of marriage (see Table 3.10, Model 1). Compared with women who earned less than 2,000,000 yen per year, those who earned greater than or equal to 4,000,000 yen per year yielded a 3.4 times greater risk of marriage. Likewise, the hazard rate of marriage was 3.4 times higher for women who earned 3,000,000–3,990,000 yen per year. According to the new home economics theory, high earning power in women should result in a low probability of marriage by a reduction in the gains from marriage. Yet, as shown in Table 3.10, the reverse is the case; since high earning power in women serves to enhance the

Table 3.10 Results of latent class event-history analysis for women

	Model 1	Model 2	Model 3	Model 4	Model 5	Model 6
Covariate	Coefficient	Coefficient	Coefficient	Coefficient	Coefficient	Coefficient
Constant	−3.76***	−3.67***	−3.71***	−4.37***	−5.06***	−3.20***
Women's age+						
Under 24	0.19	0.12	0.33	0.23	0.87	0.32
25–29	0.87	0.87	0.95	0.89	0.37	0.94
(30–34)						
Over 35	1.66*	1.54*	1.30*	1.64*	0.91*	1.17*
Birth cohort						
Before 1969	−2.52**	−2.49**	−2.05**	−2.42**	−2.54*	−1.92**
(1970–1974)						
1975–1979	0.84	0.84	0.76	0.89	1.28	0.69
After 1980	1.19	1.17	0.83	1.20	1.50	0.77
Birth order						
First daughter	0.57	0.53	0.40	0.56		
(Other)						
Co-residence with parents+						
Yes	−0.44	−0.52				
(No)						
Women's income+						
(Less than 2,000,000 yen)						
2,000,000–2,990,000 yen	0.79**		0.72**	0.84**	0.93*	0.67**
3,000,000–3,990,000 yen	1.48***		1.28***	1.52***	1.42*	1.20***
4,000,000 yen–	1.24*		1.30**	1.37**	1.79*	1.25**
Women's occupation+						
(Out of employment)						
Professional/managerial		1.18**				
Clerical/sales/service		1.08**				
Manual/agriculture/other		0.76				
Cohabitation experience before marriage+						
Yes			0.84**	0.69**		
(No)						
Premarital pregnancy+						
Yes	1.53***	1.53***		1.50***		
(No)						

(continued)

Table 3.10 (continued)

	Model 1	Model 2	Model 3	Model 4	Model 5	Model 6
Covariate	Coefficient	Coefficient	Coefficient	Coefficient	Coefficient	Coefficient
Latent class						
(Neutral)						
Conservative					1.45	
Progressive					−2.66*	
Log likelihood	−702.83	−706.61	−695.42	−653.43	−642.45	−705.20
BIC	179.84	180.16	177.44	169.68	179.46	174.82
N	358	358	358	358	358	358

Reference categories in parentheses
+ is a time-varying covariate
Time-varying variables take values prior to the occurrence of an event
*$p < 0.10$; **$p < 0.05$; ***$p < 0.01$
Source The Japanese Generations and Gender Survey

economic viability of married life, women with higher salaries may be more likely to marry than women with lower incomes.

Interestingly, co-residence with parents does not have a significant effect on female entry into marriage, although living in the parental home bears a significant affect on males when it comes to marriage. In an analysis of Japanese marriage, it is found that women living with their parents delay the transition to marriage when they perform only a small amount of domestic work in their parental home (Raymo 2003b; Raymo and Ono 2007). This finding suggests that the amount of household work to be performed, rather than co-residence itself, plays an essential role in these women's entry into marriage. With this point in mind, it is arguable that the contrasting outcomes of co-residence with parents upon men and women are attributable in part to the contrasting amount of domestic work expected of each gender. To be specific, since unmarried sons hardly ever perform domestic work when they live with parents in Japan, living with parents is favourable for these men. By contrast, unmarried daughters are to some extent forced to perform domestic work, while they live at home with their parents. Because of this, co-residence with parents has a significant effect on whether and when males marry, but does not have a significant effect on females' entry into marriage. In short, co-residence with parents is not as advantageous for women as it is for men.

As is the case with men, birth order does not affect women's marriage significantly. If the maintenance of a family line is still important in Japanese society, a first child will be encouraged to marry earlier than a second or third child. Yet, neither sons' nor daughters' birth order affects the risk of marriage. It hence follows that the consciousness of maintaining a family line is weak in contemporary Japan.

With reference to female occupation, the "professional" and "clerical" categories yield a large risk of marriage (see Table 3.10, Model 2). For instance, the hazard rate of marriage was 2.5 times greater for women engaged in a professional job than those who were out of employment. The reason for the difference in the occupational effect appears to follow along similar lines with the case for income.

More specifically, since a professional or a managerial job makes marriage more economically viable, women in these jobs exhibit a greater marriage probability.

Models 3 and 4 of Table 3.10 were provided to examine the influence of cohabitation on marriage. First of all, the experience of cohabitation increases a risk of marriage significantly. Compared with women who had ever experienced cohabitation, those who had not experienced it produced a hazard rate of marriage 2.3 times greater (see Table 3.10, Model 3). Interestingly, the experience of cohabitation is still statistically significant in Model 4 of Table 3.10, which includes premarital pregnancy as a covariate. In the case of men, when premarital pregnancy was included in the model, cohabitation experience changed from significant to insignificant. Yet, such a change is not seen in the case of women. In other words, even with the effect of a premarital conception controlled, cohabitation encourages female marriage. In this regard, the entry into cohabitation itself may be a prelude to marriage for women, with no relation to premarital pregnancy.

Finally, we will examine the effect of ideational factors on marriage behaviour. As shown in Model 5 of Table 3.10, progressive attitudes significantly reduce a risk of marriage. Compared with women of neutral attitudes, those with progressive attitudes had an approximately 90 % lower hazard rate of marriage. We can therefore argue that ideational factors affect female marriage behaviour. We should not, however, overlook that the goodness of fit is not much improved in Model 5, compared with Model 6 excluding attitudinal variables. Indeed, the value of BIC is not smaller in Model 5 than in Model 6 of Table 3.10, although the log-likelihood ratio test shows that the two models are significantly different from each other. Thus, it follows that the influence of ideational factors on female marriage is relatively weak.

3.8 A Change in the Attitudes of Unmarried People

In the previous section, we investigated the relation between attitudes and marriage behaviour. We should not, however, overlook a reverse relation between these two factors. As Elster (1983) points out, experiencing a life-changing event or encountering an awkward situation may affect an individual consciousness. Thus, it is possible that the transition to marriage changes attitudes towards partnership and family. Indeed, it is pointed out that young adults' commitment to traditional family values is weakened by cohabitation and other non-traditional lifestyles (Axinn and Thornton 1992; Waite et al. 1986). It is therefore necessary to investigate the impact of a life event on an ideational change. In the following sections, we will examine the influence of marriage on attitudes.

Table 3.11 displays respondents' attitudes between the first and third waves of the JGGS. First of all, men's attitudes are, as a whole, not so consistent between the first and the third wave. Cramer's coefficient of association was below 0.25 for opinion Items (a), (c) and (e) of the table, which indicates that the strength

Table 3.11 Value-orientations between the 1st wave and the 3rd wave (%)

Husbands	3rd wave				Wives	3rd wave			
1st wave	Agree	Uncertain	Disagree	*N*	1st wave	Agree	Uncertain	Disagree	*N*
(a) *The main purpose of marriage is to have children*									
Agree	52.8	41.5	5.7	53	Agree	48.1	40.4	11.5	52
Uncertain	26.5	61.2	12.2	147	Uncertain	14.6	68.2	17.2	151
Disagree	15.2	57.6	27.3	66	Disagree	13.6	50.3	36.1	155
N	77	150	39	266	*N*	68	202	88	358
Cramer's coefficient of association: 0.23					Cramer's coefficient of association: 0.26				
(b) *It is all right for a man and woman to live together without being married*									
Agree	69.7	22.7	7.6	132	Agree	69.1	18.9	12.0	217
Uncertain	43.8	40.0	16.3	80	Uncertain	37.6	47.3	15.1	93
Disagree	27.8	29.6	42.6	54	Disagree	25.0	39.6	35.4	48
N	142	78	46	266	*N*	197	104	57	358
Cramer's coefficient of association: 0.30					Cramer's coefficient of association: 0.28				
(c) *It is much better for everyone if the man earns the main living and the woman takes care of the home and family*									
Agree	48.0	48.0	4.1	73	Agree	46.3	40.3	13.4	67
Uncertain	28.6	54.9	16.5	133	Uncertain	21.6	58.8	19.6	153
Disagree	15.0	46.7	38.3	60	Disagree	11.6	40.6	47.8	138
N	82	136	48	266	*N*	80	173	105	358
Cramer's coefficient of association: 0.25					Cramer's coefficient of association: 0.28				
(d) *Parents should provide financial help for their adult children when the children are having financial difficulties*									
Agree	43.4	49.4	7.2	83	Agree	35.1	56.4	8.5	94
Uncertain	22.6	59.4	18.1	133	Uncertain	23.3	59.3	17.5	189
Disagree	18.0	32.0	50.0	100	Disagree	12.0	44.0	44.0	75
N	75	136	55	266	*N*	86	198	74	358
Cramer's coefficient of association: 0.29					Cramer's coefficient of association: 0.26				
(e) *A man can have a full and satisfying life without marrying*					(f) *A woman can have a full and satisfying life without marrying*				
Agree	41.2	42.4	16.5	85	Agree	56.0	35.5	8.5	141
Uncertain	25.0	57.1	17.9	140	Uncertain	26.0	59.7	14.3	154
Disagree	26.8	34.2	39.0	41	Disagree	19.1	39.7	41.3	63
N	81	130	55	266	*N*	131	167	60	358
Cramer's coefficient of association: 0.18					Cramer's coefficient of association: 0.30				

The sum of cells in each row is 100 %
Source The Japanese Generations and Gender Survey

of connection between attitudes of the first and the third wave is not so strong. In particular, men's attitudes fluctuate in Item (e). For instance, 42.4 % of men who agreed that a man can have a full and satisfying life without marrying in the first wave moved to the "uncertain" category, while 16.5 % of them shifted to the "disagree" category. Only 41.2 % of the male respondents stayed within the same answering category for opinion Item (e). Women's attitudes also do not remain much stable between the two waves of the survey. Indeed, Cramer's coefficient of association stands at about 0.30 for all items, which indicates the connection of attitudes between the first and the third wave is relatively mild. To take a typical case, 56.0 % of women who agreed with the opinion Item (f) in the first wave still stayed within the same category in the third wave. Likewise, 59.7 % of the female respondents held on in the "Uncertain" category in both waves.

In order to examine the differential tendency between men' and women's attitudes in detail, Graph 3.12 displays a trajectory of latent classes from the first to the third wave of the survey. As shown in Graph 3.12, men's latent classes change very saliently. More specifically, the proportion of the neutral group declined between years 2004 and 2010, whereas the size of the conservative and the progressive groups increased during the same period. In fact, the percentage for the

Graph. 3.12 Trajectory of latent class **a** Men, **b** Women. *Source* The Japanese Generations and Gender Survey

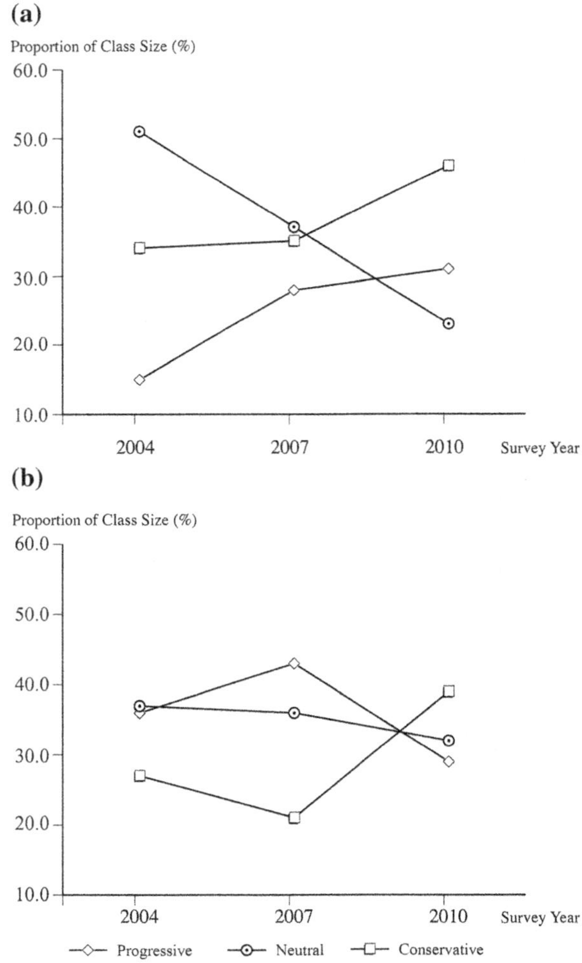

neutral class considerably fell from 51.0 % in 2004 to 22.9 % in 2010, while that of the progressive class rose steeply from 15.0 to 30.9 % in the same period. Moreover, the size of the conservative group also increased from 34.0 % in the first survey to 46.2 % in the third survey. On the other hand, women's class size shows a relatively mild change (see Graph 3.12). Their size of the neutral class remained almost unchanged between years 2004 and 2010. Furthermore, the percentage of the conservative group rose only from 15.0 % in the first survey to 17.1 % in the third survey. In contrast, the percentage for the progressive group showed a mild decline from 27.0 % in 2004 to 39.4 % in 2010, although it temporarily rose to 43.1 % in 2007. Hence, we may argue that attitudes towards partnership and family are more stable for women than for men.

3.9 Results of the Logistic Latent Class Analysis of Marriage

In order to investigate the influence of marriage on attitudes, we will conduct a logistic latent class analysis (Hagenaars and McCutcheon 2002) in this section. This analysis is expressed in the following way.

$$\log\left[\frac{\pi_{i|j}}{1-\pi_{i|j}}\right] = \alpha + \sum \beta_k x_{ikt} \tag{3.4}$$

Here, $\pi_{i|j}$ is the probability of an individual i belonging to a latent class j; α is a constant term; x_{ikt} is a manifest independent variable x_k of an individual i at t wave; and β_k is a parameter of the variable. All models in the present analysis have random intercepts and random-effect coefficients.

Table 3.12 displays the results of analysis for men. First of all, younger birth cohorts tend to have more neutral attitudes to marriage and family (see Table 3.12, Model 1). This trend is particularly conspicuous in the two birth cohorts of the 1970s. For instance, the odds ratio for neutral over progressive attitudes was 23 times greater for the 1975–1979 birth cohort than for the cohort before 1969. Yet, the birth cohorts do not show a significant coefficient in the odds ratio for conservative over progressive attitudes. Hence, it follows that only the proportion of men who have neutral attitudes increases, as their birth cohort becomes younger. By contrast, men's age does not exert a clear effect on either the odds ratio for neutral over progressive attitudes or the odds ratio for conservative over progressive attitudes. Only men over age 35 significantly decrease the ratio of neutral over progressive attitudes. This result indicates that men's attitudes towards marriage and family are hardly affected by their age.

As for men's income, only the highest income group exerts a significant effect on their attitudes. More specifically, neither the odds ratio for neutral over progressive attitudes nor the odds ratio for conservative over progressive attitudes displayed any differences in the "less than 2,000,000 yen", the "2,000,000–2,990,000

Table 3.12 Results of latent class logistic analysis for men

	Model 1		Model 2		Model 3		Model 4		Model 5	
	Neutral/ progressive	Conservative/ progressive	Neutral/ progressive	Conservative/ progressive	Neutral/ progressive	Conservative/ progressive	Neutral/ progressive	Conservative/ progressive	Neutral/ progressive	Conservative/ progressive
Covariate	Coefficient	Coefficient	Coefficient	Coefficient	Coefficient	Coefficient	Coefficient	Coefficient	Coefficient	Coefficient
Constant	−3.99**	−1.56*	−3.42***	−1.62*	−2.84*	−0.47**	−3.60**	−0.59**	−3.52**	−0.31*
Men's age+										
Under 24	1.70	−0.37	1.80	−0.32	1.53	−0.42	1.48	−0.36	1.48	−0.37
(25–29)										
30–34	0.06	0.74	−0.16	0.80	0.07	0.69	0.04	0.73	0.03	0.73
Over 35	−1.51*	−0.32	−1.63*	−0.30	−1.13*	−0.18	−1.03*	−0.07	−1.07*	−0.06
Birth cohort										
(Before 1969)										
1970–1974	3.04***	1.23	3.37***	1.73	3.09**	1.07	2.98**	0.91	3.01***	0.89
1975–1979	3.14***	1.19	3.53***	1.64	3.49***	1.22	3.59***	1.00	3.59***	0.97
After 1980	1.70**	−0.53	1.45***	−0.25	1.47**	−0.51	1.41**	−0.55	1.40**	−0.55
Birth order										
First son	0.71	0.03	0.74	0.17	0.74	0.05	0.74	0.05	0.69	0.04
(Other)										
Co-residence with parents+										
Yes	2.08	0.88	1.82	0.65						
(No)										

(continued)

Table 3.12 (continued)

	Model 1		Model 2		Model 3		Model 4		Model 5	
	Neutral/ progressive	Conservative/ progressive	Neutral/ progressive	Conservative/ progressive	Neutral/ progressive	Conservative/ progressive	Neutral/ progressive	Conservative/ progressive	Neutral/ progressive	Conservative/ progressive
Covariate	Coefficient	Coefficient	Coefficient	Coefficient	Coefficient	Coefficient	Coefficient	Coefficient	Coefficient	Coefficient
Men's income+										
Less than 2,000,000 yen	0.19	−0.10			0.14	−0.16	0.19	−0.12	0.22	−0.11
2,000,000–2,990,000 yen	0.93	0.35			0.83	0.29	0.87	0.31	0.91	0.32
(3,000,000–3,990,000 yen)										
4,000,000 yen –	0.50	1.23***			0.69	1.41**	0.46	1.18**	0.51	1.20**
Men's occupation+										
Out of employment			0.99	0.18						
Professional/ managerial			1.34**	0.78*						
(Clerical/ sales/service)										
Manual/ agriculture/ other			0.92	0.67						

(continued)

Table 3.12 (continued)

	Model 1		Model 2		Model 3		Model 4		Model 5	
	Neutral/ progressive	Conservative/ progressive	Neutral/ progressive	Conservative/ progressive	Neutral/ progressive	Conservative/ progressive	Neutral/ progressive	Conservative/ progressive	Neutral/ progressive	Conservative/ progressive
Covariate	Coefficient	Coefficient	Coefficient	Coefficient	Coefficient	Coefficient	Coefficient	Coefficient	Coefficient	Coefficient
Cohabitation experience before marriage+										
Yes					−0.69**	−0.99**				
(No)										
Marital status+										
Married							0.52	0.40		
(Not married)										
Marriage type+										
Pregnancy-dependent marriage									3.03*	−0.43
(Marriage)										
Not married									−0.15	−0.28
Log likelihood	−1890.86		−1894.50		−1890.61		−1934.31		−1891.19	
BIC	4152.12		4159.40		4151.62		4131.49		4164.74	
N	266		266		266		266		266	

Reference categories in parentheses
+ is a time-varying covariate
$*p < 0.10$; $**p < 0.05$; $***p < 0.01$
Source The Japanese Generations and Gender Survey

yen", and the "3,000,000–3,990,000 yen" groups. Yet, the odds ratio for conservative over progressive attitudes was 3.4 times greater for men who earned greater than or equal to 4,000,000 yen a year than for those who earned 3,000,000–3,990,000 yen. Thus, we may argue that men with very high salaries tend to have conservative attitudes towards marriage and family. Birth order does not have a significant impact on men's attitudes. Likewise, co-residence with parents does not exercise a significant influence on their attitudes. It therefore follows that these family-related factors have no bearing on men's attitudes.

Model 2 of Table 3.12 was conducted to examine the impact of occupation on attitudes. The overall impression is that men's attitudes are not so clearly different between their occupations. It should nevertheless be noted that men who are engaged in a professional or a managerial job are less progressive. The odds ratio for neutral over progressive attitudes was 3.8 times greater in the "professional category" than in the "clerical" category. Similarly, compared with men in a clerical job, those in a professional job produced a 2.2 times greater odds ratio for conservative over progressive attitudes. As far as this result shows, the proportion of men with progressive attitudes is significantly lower when they work in a professional or a managerial occupation. In other words, men in the upper class tend to have conservative values towards partnership and family relations.

With regard to cohabitation, when men experience cohabitation, they become progressive in their attitudes (see Table 3.12, Model 3). Indeed, the odds ratio for conservative over progressive attitudes was 63 % lower for men who had ever cohabited than for those who had not cohabited. Likewise, ever-cohabited men yielded a 50 % smaller odds ratio for neutral over progressive attitudes than never-cohabited men. We can therefore argue that men hold progressive attitudes towards marriage and family when they experience cohabitation before marriage.

Finally, we will examine the impact of marriage in Models 4 and 5 of Table 3.12. As seen in Model 4 of this table, marriage does not, as a whole, exercise a significant effect on men's attitudes. Yet, the impact of marriage differs between the types of marriage (see Table 3.12, Model 5). Compared to men who married without a premarital pregnancy, men with a pregnancy-dependent marriage produced a 21 times greater odds ratio for neutral over progressive attitudes. We may therefore argue that when men are triggered to marry due to a premarital pregnancy, their attitudes towards marriage and family become ambivalent. When their marriage is not, however, accompanied by a premarital pregnancy, their experience of marriage does not affect their attitudes.

Now, let us turn to women's analysis in Table 3.13. The first noticeable point is that birth cohorts do not show a significant effect on women's attitudes (see Table 3.13, Model 1). This clearly contrasts with the case for men, in which a salient influence was found between birth cohorts. On the other hand, age groups exert a relatively clear influence on female attitudes. Admittedly, compared with women under age 24, those aged between 30 and 34 produced a seven times greater odds ratio for neutral over progressive attitudes significantly. Similarly, the 25–29 age group yields a significant odds ratio of conservative over progressive

Table 3.13 Results of latent class logistic analysis for women

	Model 1		Model 2		Model 3		Model 4		Model 5	
	Neutral/ progressive	Conservative/ progressive	Neutral/ progressive	Conservative/ progressive	Neutral/ progressive	Conservative/ progressive	Neutral/ progressive	Conservative/ progressive	Neutral/ progressive	Conservative/ progressive
Covariate	Coefficient	Coefficient	Coefficient	Coefficient	Coefficient	Coefficient	Coefficient	Coefficient	Coefficient	Coefficient
Constant	−2.23**	−0.92**	−2.56**	−1.63**	−1.29**	−1.04**	−1.88**	−0.77**	−2.35*	−1.06*
Women's age+										
(Under 24)										
25–29	1.02**	0.75**	1.07**	0.52*	1.07**	0.74**	1.08**	0.78**	1.06**	0.77*
30–34	1.94***	0.80	1.84***	1.23	2.00***	0.78	2.03***	0.87	2.02***	0.86
Over 35	2.99	1.58	2.85	1.59	3.10	1.55	3.14	1.67	3.13	1.66
Birth cohort										
(Before 1969)										
1970–1974	0.38	−0.14	0.47	−0.25	0.41	−0.14	0.46	−0.09	0.46	−0.08
1975–1979	0.95	0.48	1.12	0.45	1.06	0.56	1.12	0.60	1.13	0.61
After 1980	1.11	1.05	1.04	1.41	1.24	1.13	1.32	1.22	1.32	1.23
Birth order										
First daughter	0.33	0.65	0.29	0.44	0.32	0.65	0.32	0.64	0.30	0.64
(Other)										
Co-residence with parents+										
Yes	0.56	0.28	0.42	0.71						
(No)										

(continued)

Table 3.13 (continued)

	Model 1		Model 2		Model 3		Model 4		Model 5	
	Neutral/ progressive	Conservative/ progressive	Neutral/ progressive	Conservative/ progressive	Neutral/ progressive	Conservative/ progressive	Neutral/ progressive	Conservative/ progressive	Neutral/ progressive	Conservative/ progressive
Covariate	Coefficient	Coefficient	Coefficient	Coefficient	Coefficient	Coefficient	Coefficient	Coefficient	Coefficient	Coefficient
Women's income+										
Less than 2,000,000 yen	−0.36	−0.16			−0.34	−0.14	−0.37	−0.17	−0.39	−0.17
(2,000,000–2,990,000 yen)										
3,000,000–3,990,000 yen	−0.06	−0.69			−0.04	−0.64	−0.04	−0.63	−0.03	−0.63
4,000,000 yen–	−1.11**	−1.32***			−1.13***	−1.39**	−1.13**	−1.29**	−1.13**	−1.29**
Women's occupation+										
Out of employment			−1.63	−0.02						
Professional/ managerial			−0.54*	−0.68*						
(Clerical/ sales/service)										
Manual/ agriculture/ other			−2.12	−1.23						
Cohabitation experience before marriage+										
Yes					−0.56**	−1.83				
(No)										

(continued)

Table 3.13 (continued)

	Model 1		Model 2		Model 3		Model 4		Model 5	
	Neutral/ progressive	Conservative/ progressive	Neutral/ progressive	Conservative/ progressive	Neutral/ progressive	Conservative/ progressive	Neutral/ progressive	Conservative/ progressive	Neutral/ progressive	Conservative/ progressive
Covariate	Coefficient	Coefficient	Coefficient	Coefficient	Coefficient	Coefficient	Coefficient	Coefficient	Coefficient	Coefficient
Marital status+										
Married							0.33	0.47		
(Not married)										
Marriage type+										
Pregnancy-dependent marriage									1.07	0.29
(Marriage)										
Not married									−0.03	0.46
Log likelihood	−2060.99		−2061.73		−2060.44		−2061.02		−2060.91	
BIC	4448.42		4449.91		4447.34		4448.50		4460.37	
N	358		358		358		358		358	

Reference categories in parentheses
+ is a time-varying covariate
$^*p < 0.10$; $^{**}p < 0.05$; $^{***}p < 0.01$
Source The Japanese Generations and Gender Survey

attitudes. Hence, it follows that women's age has a mild impact on their attitudes towards partnership and family relation.

As for women's earning power, a significant coefficient was identified in only the highest income group. More specifically, the odds ratio for conservative over progressive attitudes was 75 % lower for women who earned greater than or equal to 4,000,000 yen a year than for those who earned between 2,000,000 and 2,990,000 yen a year. Likewise, the "4,000,000 yen–" group yielded a 63 % lower odds ratio for neutral over progressive attitudes than the "2,000,000–2,990,000" group. These results indicate that women with extremely high salaries hold more progressive attitudes to partnership and family relations.

The coefficient of birth order is statistically insignificant, so that attitudes are not different between first daughters and other daughters. Similarly, co-residence with parents has no significant effect on women's attitudes.

Model 2 of Table 3.13 was provided to investigate the impact of occupation. The overall impression of the results is that women's attitudes are not so discernibly different between their occupations. Only professional and managerial jobs show a significant effect, and women working in these occupations produced a 50 % lower odds ratio for conservative over progressive attitudes than those working in clerical or sales occupations. Likewise, the odds ratio for neutral over progressive attitudes is significantly small. These findings indicate that professional and managerial women are relatively progressive.

In terms of cohabitation, its experience shows a mild impact on female attitudes (see Table 3.13, Model 3). Although the odds ratio for conservative over progressive attitudes is statistically insignificant, the odds ratio for neutral over progressive attitudes is 43 % lower with statistical significance for ever-cohabited women than never-cohabited women. We can therefore argue that, only if women had ambiguous attitudes before marriage, they become more progressive after cohabitation.

Finally, we will examine the influence of marriage. As in the case with men's attitudes, women's attitudes do not change whether or not they are being married (see Table 3.13, Model 4). It follows that the experience of marriage has no substantial impact on female attitudes. Furthermore, types of marriage also exercise no significant effect on attitudes (see Table 3.13, Model 5). As shown in Table 3.12, men who married due to a premarital pregnancy tended to have ambivalent attitudes. Yet, such a tendency is not observed in the case of women. In Model 5 of Table 3.13, there is no difference in attitudes between women whose marriage is set off by a premarital pregnancy and women who marry without being pregnant before marriage. In other words, whichever type of marriage women experience, it does not change female attitudes to marriage and family.

3.10 Conclusion

Since the latter half of the 1970s, Japanese age at marriage has started to rise in tandem with a decline in the proportion of people ever-married. As mentioned before, mean age at first marriage for men and women stood at nearly age thirty in 2012. In addition, dependent marriages, cohabitations and divorces have increased in number. These phenomena have gradually manifested themselves in Japan since the 1980s.

Looking at Japanese society from a broad perspective, we can recognize that women's socio-economic circumstances have changed drastically over the past few decades. The number of women engaged in gainful employment has increased in tandem with a rise in the percentage of women going to college or university. Although the faltering financial climate after the economic bubble of the 1980s suppressed the pace of this change, the economic empowerment of Japanese women still continues to expand. In addition, as far as some national opinion surveys show, people's attitudes towards family and lifestyle have also changed during the same period.

The main purpose of this chapter was to investigate the influence of economic and ideational factors on marriage behaviour in Japan. The results of the analysis, first of all, suggest that economic factors have a powerful impact on marriage in Japan. In concrete terms, men and women with a high level of income tended to get married with a greater probability than those with a lower level of income. Furthermore, people engaged in a professional or a managerial job also were more likely to enter into marriage.

Second, the findings of this chapter indicate that ideational factors, at the same time, affect marriage behaviour in Japan, although their effects were not so strong. To be specific, less traditional and more self-centred attitudes reduced a risk of male marriage. Likewise, the probability of women's entry into marriage was decreased in tandem with the strengthening of both progressive and individualistic attitudes. It can therefore be concluded that Japanese marriage behaviour is affected by both economic and ideational factors, but the extent of influence is greater for the former than the latter.

Third, it was, in our analysis, suggested that economic factors have an influence on attitudes towards partnership and family. While men with very high income tended to have more conservative attitudes, high-salaried women's attitudes were more progressive. Hence, it follows that an earning power has a different influence on attitudes between men and women.

Fourth, the results of the present analysis suggest that the experience of cohabitation changes one's attitudes, but the experience of marriage, regardless of marriage types, hardly affects one's attitudes. More specifically, ever-cohabited men and women tended to have progressive attitudes than those never-cohabited. Thus, it is likely that attitudes to partnership and family formation become more progressive as more Japanese adults experience cohabitation. In contrast, people's attitudes were almost the same, regardless of marital status and marriage types.

This tendency is particularly clear for women. Taking the above results into consideration, we can conclude that economic and ideational factors affect Japanese marriage behaviour, but marriage does not exert an influence on the values and attitudes of Japanese people.

References

Anderson, K. H., & Hill, M. A. (1983). Marriage and labor market discrimination in Japan. *Southern Economic Journal, 49*, 941–953.

Ariès, P. (1980). Two successive motivations for the declining birth rate in the west. *Population and Development Review, 6*, 645–650.

Axinn, W. G., & Thornton, A. (1992). The relationship between cohabitation and divorce: Selectivity or causal influence? *Demography, 29*, 357–374.

Becker, G. S. (1975). *Human capital: A theoretical and empirical analysis, with special reference to education*. Chicago: University of Chicago Press.

Billari, F., & Rosina, A. (2004). Italian "Latest-Late" transition to adulthood: An exploration of its consequences on fertility. *Genus, 60*, 71–87.

Bongaarts, J., & Potter, R. G. (1983). *Fertility, biology and behavior: An analysis of the proximate determinants*. New York: Academic Press.

Brinton, M. C. (1993). *Women and the economic miracle: Gender and work in the postwar Japan*. Berkeley: University of California Press.

Burgess, S., Propper, C., & Aassve, A. (2003). The role of income in marriage and divorce transitions among young Americans. *Journal of Population Economics, 16*, 455–475.

Caldwell, J. C. (1982). *Theory of fertility decline*. New York: Academic Press.

Carter, H., & Glick, P. C. (1976). *Marriage and divorce: A social and economic study*. Cambridge, Massachusetts: Harvard University Press.

Cherline, A. J. (1992). *Marriage, divorce, remarriage*. Cambridge, Massachusetts: Harvard University Press.

Cigno, A. (1991). *Economics of the family*. Oxford: Oxford University Press.

Coleman, D. (1993). Britain in Europe: International and regional comparisons of fertility levels and trends. In M. Ní Bhrolcháin (Ed.), *New perspectives of fertility in Britain* (pp. 67–94). London: OPCS.

Coleman, D., & Salt, J. (1992). *The British Population: Patterns, Trends, and Processes*. Oxford: Oxford University Press.

Dore, R. P. (1953). Japanese rural fertility: Some social and economic factors. *Population Studies, 7*, 62–88.

Easterlin, R. A. (1987). *Birth and fortune*. Chicago: University of Chicago Press.

Elder, G. H. (1977). *Children of the great depression: Social change in life experience*. Chicago: University of Chicago Press.

Eldridge, S., & Kiernan, K. (1985). Declining first marriage rates in England and Wales: A change in timing or a rejection of marriage? *European Journal of Population, 1*, 327–345.

Elster, J. (1983). *Sour grapes: Studies in the subversion of rationality*. Cambridge: Cambridge University Press.

Ermisch, J. (1981). Economic opportunities, marriage squeezes and the propensity to marry. *Population Studies, 35*, 347–356.

Ermisch, J. (2003). *An economic analysis of the family*. Princeton: Princeton University Press.

Freiden, A. (1974). The U.S. marriage market. In T. W. Schultz (Ed.), *Economic of the family* (pp. 352–371). Chicago: University of Chicago Press.

Gabrielli, G., & Hoem, J. M. (2010). Italy's non-negligible cohabitational unions. *European Journal of Population, 26*, 33–46.

Giele, J. Z., & Elder, G. H. (1998). *Methods of life course research: Qualitative and quantitative approaches*. Thousand Oaks, California: Sage Publications.
Goldscheider, F. K., & Waite, L. J. (1986). Sex differences in the entry into marriage. *American Journal of Sociology, 92*, 91–109.
Goode, W. J. (1963). *World revolution and family patterns*. New York: The Free Press.
Guo, S., & Fraser, M. W. (2014). *Propensity score analysis: Statistical methods and applications*. Thousand Oaks, California: Sage Publications.
Gutiérrez-Domènech, M. (2008). The impact of the labour market on the timing of marriage and births in Spain. *Journal of Population Economics, 21*, 83–110.
Hagenaars, J. A. (1993). *Loglinear models with latent variables*. Thousand Oaks, California: Sage Publications.
Hagenaars, J. A., & McCutcheon, A. L. (2002). *Applied latent class analysis*. Cambridge: Cambridge University Press.
Hajnal, J. (1965). European marriage pattern in perspective. In D. V. Glass & D. E. C. Eversley (Eds.), *Population in history: Essays in historical demography* (pp. 101–143). London: Arnold.
Hajnal, J. (1983). Two kinds of pre-industrial household formation system. In R. Wall, J. Robin & P. Laslett (Eds.), *Family forms in historic Europe* (pp. 65–104). Cambridge: Cambridge University Press.
Iacovou, M., & Parisi, L. (2009). Leaving home. In M. Brynin & J. Ermisch (Eds.), *Changing relationships* (pp. 59–72). New York: Routledge.
Kalmijn, M. (2011). The influence of men's income and employment on marriage and cohabitation: Testing Oppenheimer's theory in Europe. *European Journal of Population, 27*, 269–293.
Kiernan, K. (1996). Partnership behaviour in Europe: Recent trends and issues. In D. Coleman (Ed.), *Europe's population in the 1990s* (pp. 62–91). Oxford: Oxford University Press.
Kiernan, K. (1999). Cohabitation in Western Europe. *Population Trends, 96*, 23–32.
Kiernan, K. (2000). European perspectives on union formation. In L. J. Waite (Ed.), *The ties that bind: Perspectives on* marriage *and cohabitation* (pp. 40–58). New York: Aldine de Gruyter.
Kiernan, K. (2001). The rise of cohabitation and childbearing outside marriage in Western Europe. *International Law, Policy and the Family, 15*, 1–21.
Kiernan, K. (2002). Cohabitation in Western Europe: Trends, issues, and implications. In A. Booth & A. C. Crouter (Eds.), *Just living together: Implications of cohabitation on families, children, and social policy* (pp. 3–31). Mahwah, New Jersey: Lawrence Erlbaum Associates.
Kiernan, K. (2004a). Cohabitation and divorce across nations and generations. In P. L. Chase-Lansdale, K. Kiernan & R. J. Friedman (Eds.), *Human development across lives and generations: The potential for change* (pp. 139–170). New York: Cambridge University Press.
Kiernan, K. (2004b). Unmarried cohabitation and parenthood in Britain and Europe. *Journal of Law and Policy, 26*, 33–55.
Langbein, L. I., & Lichtman, A. J. (1978). *Ecological inference*. London: SAGE.
Lesthaeghe, R. (1983). A century of demographic and cultural change in Western Europe. *Population and Development Review, 9*, 411–436.
Lesthaeghe, R., & Meekers, D. (1986). Value changes and the dimension of familism in the European Community. *European Journal of Population, 2*, 225–268.
Lesthaeghe, R., & Surkyn, J. (1988). Cultural dynamics and economic theories of fertility change. *Population and Development Review, 14*, 1–45.
Lesthaeghe, R. (1995). The second demographic transition in Western countries: An interpretation. In K. O. Mason & J. An-Magritt (Eds.), *Gender and family change in industrialized countries* (pp. 17–62). Oxford: Clarendon Press.
Morgan, S. P., & Hiroshima, K. (1983). The persistence of extended family residence in Japan: Anachronism or alternative strategy. *American Sociological Review, 48*, 269–281.
Mortimer, J. T., & Shanahan, M. J. (2003). *Handbook of the life course*. Dordrecht: Kluwer Academic, Plenum Publishers.

Murphy, M. J. (1987). Differential family formation in Great Britain. *Journal of Biosocial Science, 19*, 463–481.
Murphy, M. J. (1989). Housing the people: From shortage to surplus. In H. Joshi (Ed.), *The changing population of Britain* (pp. 90–109). Oxford: Basil Blackwell.
National Institute of Population and Social Security Research. (2012). *The report on the fourteenth Japanese fertility survey in 2010*. Tokyo: National Institute of Population and Social Security Research.
OECE. (2011). *Employment outlook*. Paris: OECD.
Ogura, S., & Dekle, R. (1992). Explaining the declining fertility of Japanese women since 1970 through prefectural cohort data. *JCER Economic Journal, 22*, 46–76.
Oppenheimer, V. K. (1988). A theory of marriage timing. *American Journal of Sociology, 94*, 563–591.
Oppenheimer, V. K. (2000). The continuing importance of men's economic position in marriage formation. In L. J. Waite, C. Bachrach, M. Hindin, E. Thomson & A. Thornton (Eds.), *The ties that bind: Perspectives on marriage and cohabitation* (pp. 283–301). New York: Aldine de Gruyter.
Piotrowski, M., Kalleberg, A., & Rindfuss, R. R. (2015). Contingent work rising: Implications for the timing of marriage in Japan. *Journal of Marriage and Family, 77*, 1039–1056.
Raftery, A. E. (1995). Bayesian model selection in social research. In P. V. Marsden (Ed.), *Sociological methodology 1995* (pp. 111–163). Oxford: Basil Blackwell.
Raymo, J. M. (1998). Later marriages or fewer? Changes in the marital behavior of Japanese women. *Journal of Marriage and the Family, 60*, 1023–1034.
Raymo, J. M. (2003a). Educational attainment and the transition to first marriage among Japanese women. *Demography, 40*, 83–103.
Raymo, J. M. (2003b). Premarital living arrangements and the transition to first marriage in Japan. *Journal of Marriage and Family, 65*, 302–315.
Raymo, J. M., & Iwasawa, M. (2008). Premarital pregnancy and spouse pairing patterns in Japan. *Journal of Marriage and Family, 70*, 835–1091.
Raymo, J. M., Iwasawa, M., & Bumpass, L. L. (2004). Marital dissolution in Japan: Recent trends and differentials. *Demographic Research, 11*, 395–419.
Raymo, J. M., Iwasawa, M., & Bumpass, L. L. (2009). Cohabitation and first marriage in Japan. *Demography, 46*, 785–803.
Raymo, J. M., & Ono, H. (2007). Co-residence with parents, women's economic resources, and the transition to marriage in Japan. *Journal of Family Issues, 28*, 653–681.
Reher, D. S. (2004). Family ties in Western Europe: Persistent contrasts. In G. Dalla Zuanna & G. A. Micheli (Eds.), *Strong family and low fertility: A paradox?: New perspectives in interpreting contemporary family and reproductive behaviour* (pp. 45–76). Dordrecht: Kluwer Academic Publishers.
Retherford, R. D., Ogawa, N., & Matsukura, R. (2001). Late marriage and less marriage in Japan. *Population and Development Review, 27*, 65–102.
Robinson, W. S. (1950). Ecological correlations and the behavior of individuals. *American Journal of Sociology, 15*, 351–357.
Rosina, A., & Fraboni, R. (2004). Is marriage loosing its centrality in Italy? *Demographic Research, 11*, 149–172.
Ryder, N. B. (1965). The cohort as a concept in the study of social change. *American Sociological Review, 30*, 843–861.
Santos, F. P. (1975). The economics of marital status. In C. B. Lloyd (Ed.), *Sex, discrimination, and the division of labor* (pp. 244–269). New York: Columbia University Press.
Schofield, R. (1989). Family structure, demographic behaviour, and economic growth. In J. Walter & R. Schofield (Eds.), *Famine, disease and the social order in early modern society* (pp. 279–304). Cambridge: Cambridge University Press.
Simons, J. (1986a). Culture, economy and reproduction in contemporary Europe. In D. Coleman & R. Schofield (Eds.), *The state of population theory* (pp. 256–278). Oxford: Basil Blackwell.

Simons, J. (1986b). How conservative are British attitudes to childbearing. *Quarterly Journal of Social Affairs, 2*, 415–429.
Smith, R. M. (1981). Fertility, economy and household formation in England over three centuries. *Population Development and Review, 7*, 595–622.
Smith, R. M. (1986). Transfer incomes, risk and security. In D. Coleman and R. Schofield (Eds.), *The state of population theory* (pp. 188–211). Oxford: Basil Blackwell.
Smock, P. J. (2000). Cohabitation in the United States: An appraisal of research themes, findings, and implications. *Annual Review of Sociology, 26*, 1–20.
Sweeney, M. M. (2002). Two decades of family change: The shifting economic foundations of marriage. *American Sociological Review, 67*, 132–147.
The Institute of Statistical Mathematics. (2009). *A study of the Japanese national character*. Tokyo: The Institute of Statistical Mathematics.
The Ministry of Education, Culture, Sports, Science and Technology. (Various years). *Report on the Basic Survey of Schools*. Tokyo: The Ministry of Education, Culture, Sports, Science and Technology.
The Ministry of Health, Labour and Welfare. (2010). *Special report of vital statistics*. Tokyo: The Ministry of Health, Labour and Welfare.
The Ministry of Health, Labour and Welfare. (Various years). *Vital Statistics*. Tokyo: The Ministry of Health, Labour and Welfare.
The Ministry of Health, Labour and Welfare. (Various years). *Basic Survey on Wage Structure*. Tokyo: The Ministry of Health, Labour and Welfare.
The Ministry of Internal Affairs and Communications. (Various years). *Annual Report on Labour Force Survey*. Tokyo: The Ministry of Internal Affairs and Communications.
The Ministry of Internal Affairs and Communications. (Various years). *National Census*. Tokyo: The Ministry of Internal Affairs and Communications.
The Population Problems Research Council of the Mainich News Paper. (2000). *The Japanese population: Footsteps of the 50 post-war years*. Tokyo: The Population Problems Research Council of the Mainichi Newspaper.
Tsuya, N. O., & Bumpass, L. L. (2004). *Marriage, work, and family life in comparative perspective: Japan, South Korea, and the United States*. Honolulu: University of Hawaii Press.
van de Kaa, D. J. (1987). Europe's second demographic transition. *Population Bulletin* 42.
Vermunt, J. K. (1997). *Log-linear models for event histories*. London: Sage Publications.
Waite, L. J., Goldscheider, F. K., & Witsberger, C. (1986). Non-family living and the erosion of traditional family orientations among young adults. *American Sociological Review, 51*, 541–554.
Winegarden, C. R. (1984). Women's fertility, market and marital status: A test of the new household economics with international data. *Economica, 51*, 447–456.
Young, M., & Willmott, P. (1973). *The symmetrical family: A study of work and leisure in the London region*. London: Routledge and Kegan Paul.
Zuanna, G. D. (2004). The banquet of aeolus: A familistic interpretation of Italy's lowest low fertility. In G. Dalla Zuanna & G. A. Micheli (Eds.), *Strong family and low fertility: A paradox?: New perspectives in interpreting contemporary family and reproductive behaviour* (pp. 105–125). Dordrecht: Kluwer Academic Publishers.
Zuanna, G. D., Atoh, M., Castiglioni, M., & Kojima, K. (1998). Late marriage among young people: The case of Italy and Japan. *Genus, 54*, 187–232.

Chapter 4
Economic Change, Value Shift and Fertility Behaviour

4.1 Introduction

In this chapter, we will investigate the influence of economic and ideational factors on fertility behaviour in Japan. As discussed in Chap. 1, in demographic literature, a change in fertility patterns is sometimes related to the approximate determinants of fertility (Balbo et al. 2013; Bongaarts 1976, 1978; Davis and Black 1956). For example, Westoff and Ryder (1977) argue that the spread of the pill was the main cause of fertility decline in the USA from the late 1960s. Similarly, Murphy (1993a, b) claims that the fall in the British fertility rate in the 1960s and the 1970s was attributable to the increase of contraceptive pill users, and its further reduction in the 1980s was the result of the diffusion of sterilization.[1]

Marriage may be also regarded as one of the approximate determinants of fertility. Admittedly, it is reasoned that in a society where couples rarely practice contraception, female marriage age will be strongly linked to female level of fertility through a change in the risk of pregnancy over time. However, in a society where married couples practise effective modern contraception and prefer small family size, the level of fertility is expected to be less dependent on marriage age (Westoff et al. 1987). Accordingly, the timing of marriage should, in theory, bear little relation to the level of fertility in developed countries where effective contraception is widely practised. Prior studies indicate, nevertheless, that even in a society where fertility control is carried out extensively and effectively, a correlation between marriage and fertility is still observed (Bumpass 1969; Bumpass and Mburugu 1977; Busfield 1972), although an increase in the number of extramarital births tends to weaken this connection between the two elements. In this regard,

[1]Caution is needed when considering the relationship between fertility behaviour and contraceptive methods. Superficially, we can find the link between a change in fertility and a spread of effective contraception methods. However, explanations of this kind do not take into account the reason why such new methods have become popular as a method of contraception.

N. Fukuda, *Marriage and Fertility Behaviour in Japan*,
DOI 10.1007/978-981-10-0294-6_4

the analysis of marriage behaviour may remain a tool in understanding the patterns of childbearing indirectly.

At the same time, it should, however, be kept in mind that marriage is nothing more than an approximate determinant of fertility pattern. Admittedly, marriage behaviour examined in the previous chapter has considerably contributed to our understanding of the partnership formation in Japan, but the features of fertility behaviour are very insufficiently captured by only marriage patterns (for details, see Chap. 1). Therefore, it is necessary to investigate fertility behaviour directly in order to understand the patterns of Japanese family formation more completely.

This chapter is divided into two main parts. The first part of the chapter is dedicated to examining the influence of economic and ideational factors on fertility behaviour; we will analyse the impact of childbirth on couples' attitudes in the second part of the chapter. We will first look at Japanese fertility trends in the light of the socio-economic environments surrounding childbearing and Japanese attitudes towards children. Subsequently, we will briefly provide the theoretical background of this analysis. After explaining the data and methods used in this chapter, we will present the results of this analysis with regard to the influence of economic and ideational factors on fertility behaviour. Finally, we will investigate the impact of childbirth on couples' attitudes.

4.2 Fertility Trends in Japan

The Japanese total period fertility rate (TPFR) has declined steadily since the 1970s in tandem with a rise in the tempo of childbearing. Graph 4.1 shows the TPFR and mother's mean age at birth since 1960. The mean age by birth order in this graph is computed for all births, including extramarital births. If the proportion of extramarital births over all births is high, the mean age computed for all births cannot be regarded as an appropriate index of fertility timing for married couples. In this case, the mean age will not properly reflect the couple's birth history after marriage (Hirschman and Rindfuss 1982). As we will discuss in more detail below, since the number of extramarital and premarital births is quite small in Japan, the mean age computed for all births can be regarded as an index of the timing of childbirth for married couples.

The overall picture of Graph 4.1 shows that the Japanese TPFR has sharply fallen since the middle of the 1970s, in tandem with a rise in the age at which Japanese women have children. In concrete terms, although the TPFR remained fixed at around 2.0 until 1974, the fertility rate started to decline drastically from 1975, reaching 1.39 in 2010. As for the mean mother's age at first birth, this also remained stable at around 25.5 years of age until 1975, and then rose considerably to age 29.3 in 2010. Likewise, the age at second and third birth rose from age 28.15 in 1975 to age 31.2 in 2010, and from age 30.51 to 32.7, respectively. This evidence indicates that Japan has experienced a great decline of the TPFR, coinciding with a dramatic rise in the mean age of women's giving birth.

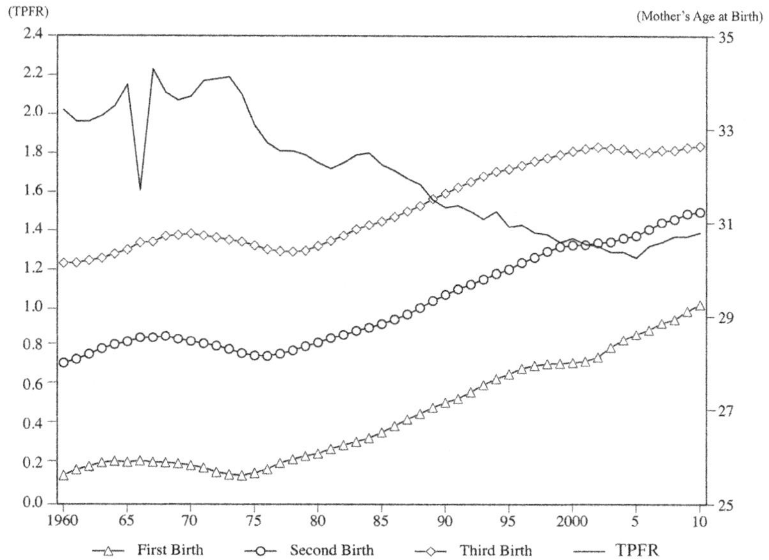

Graph 4.1 TPFR and mean age at birth in Japan since 1960. *Source* Ministry of Health, Labour and Welfare (various years). Vital statistics

Despite this fact, much caution is needed when interpreting the actual change in fertility pattern as the TPFR is strongly affected by the timing of childbearing (Bongaarts and Feeney 1998, 2000). More specifically, since the TPFR is calculated on hypothetical cohorts, it is the sum of the age-specific fertility rates at a particular point in time. Hence, the TPFR is not always equal to the number of children a woman has in her life. In other words, the TPFR's value fluctuates by rapid changes in the timing of women's childbirth. On the other hand, since completed family size or the total cohort fertility rate (TCFR) is the average number of children that women of a particular cohort actually have during their reproductive lifespan, the TCFR's value is not subject to the temporal change of childbearing. In short, if age at childbearing falls, the TPFR will overestimate the TCFR. In contrast, the TPFR will underestimate the TCFR in the case of rising age at childbearing. Therefore, in grasping a true trend of fertility pattern, it is necessary to look at cohort fertility as well as period fertility.

Graph 4.2 displays the cumulative fertility rate by female birth cohort. Since younger cohorts do not reach the end of their reproductive period, it is difficult to show the definitive trend of complete family size. Nevertheless, if we regard the cumulative fertility rate at age 40 as an index of complete family size, we can identify that the number of children born to a woman decreases after the year 1960 cohort. In concrete terms, the cumulative fertility rate at age 40 fluctuates at around 2.0 in the 1940 and 1950 birth cohorts. Yet, the rate falls from 1.8 in the 1960 birth cohort to 1.4 in the 1970 birth cohort. Since women who were born in the year 1960 reached age 30 in 1990, it follows that Japanese fertility started

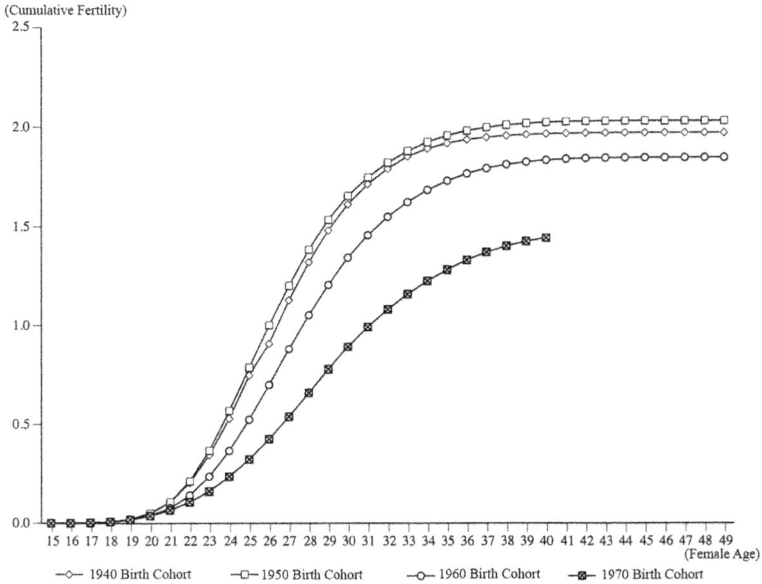

Graph 4.2 Cumulative fertility rate by birth cohort in Japan. *Source* Ministry of Health, Labour and Welfare (various years). Vital statistics

to fall after the turn of the century from a cohort perspective. On the other hand, looking at the fact that the TPFR started to decline in 1974, we can recognize that Japanese period fertility had already fallen in the latter half of the 1970s. As mentioned previously, since the TPFR is affected by a change in the timing of childbirth, we can ascertain that the drastic fall of the Japanese TPFR between the late 1970s and early 1990s was considerably attributable to the temporal change of childbearing behaviour.

When looking at characteristics of Japanese fertility patterns, we should not ignore that most babies are born in wedlock. Indeed, the proportion of out-of-wedlock births over all births is much lower in Japan than in other industrialized countries. Graph 4.3 shows the historical change in percentages of extramarital births in selected industrialized countries. The data displayed on the graph provide a first impression that the percentage of Japanese extramarital births is extremely low and stable when compared with data from the other countries. In fact, its percentage has slightly increased over the past 40 years, but still remains around 2.0 %. Italy, like Japan, had a low percentage of extramarital births until the early 1990s, but its figure has rapidly increased since the mid-1990s (Zuanna 2004). As a result, about 20 % of Italian babies were born out of wedlock in 2010. Moreover, the graphs shows that the percentage of extramarital births in the year 2010 was comprised of 32.3 % of all births in Germany, 47.1 % in UK, 55.0 % in France, and 54.2 % in Sweden. The extraordinary low percentage of Japanese out-of-wedlock births indicates that marriage is still a dominant institution for procreation in Japan. Furthermore, this feature leads us think that, at an aggregated level, an

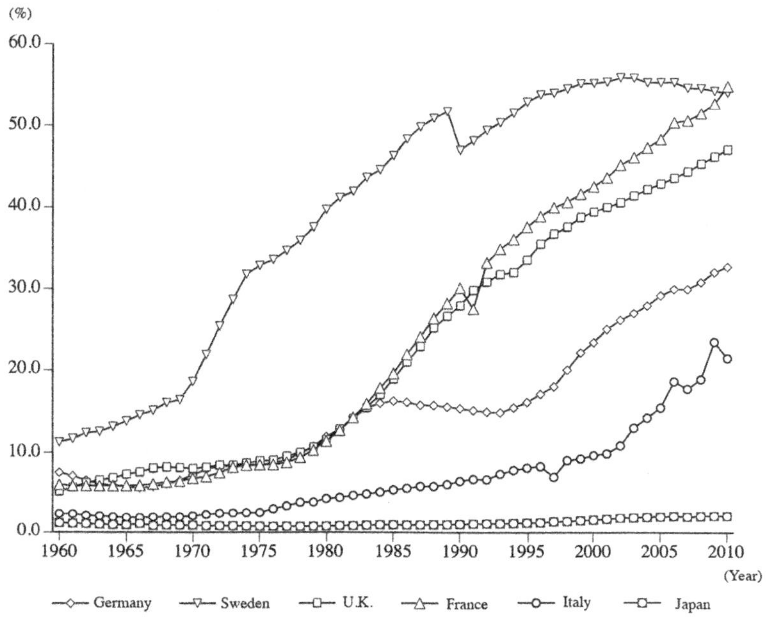

Graph 4.3 Percentages of extramarital births in selected countries. *Source* Eurostat Demographic Database http://epp.eurostat.ec.europa.eu/portal/page/portal/population/data/database. Ministry of Health, Labour and Welfare (various years). Vital statistics

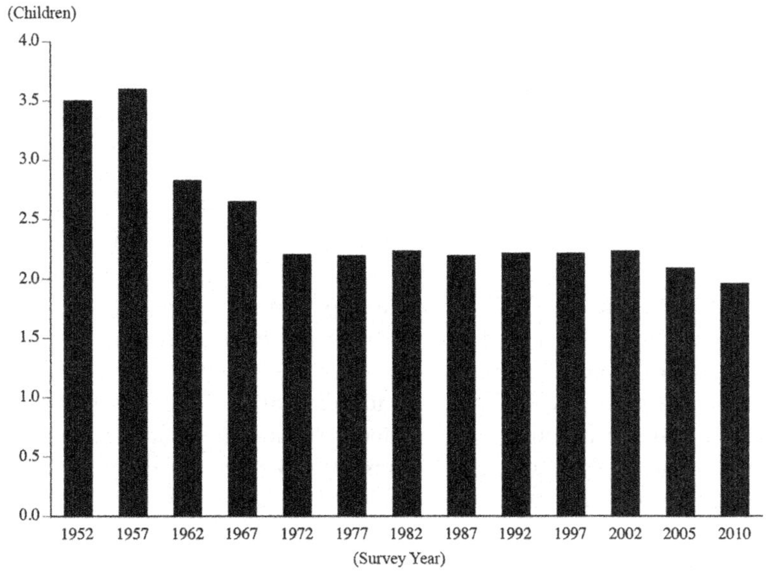

Graph 4.4 The achieved number of children for married couples in Japan. *Note* The achieved number of children is calculated for couples who have been married between 15 and 19 years. *Source* National Institute of Population and Social Security Research (various years). The Japanese National Fertility Survey

increase in the number of single people is related to a fall in the Japanese fertility rate, simply because marriages decrease in number.

We have hitherto showed the features of Japanese fertility, but the most important point to note is that the fertility behaviour of married couples has also undergone a salient change over the past few decades. As seen in Graph 4.4, recent married couples tend to have fewer children. Until the end of the 1960s, married couples who had been married between 15 and 19 years, on average, had more than 2.5 children. Yet, this figure fell to about 2.0 children in the 1970s and dropped to below 2.0 in the 2000s. As far as this evidence shows, we can argue that married couples' reproductive behaviour is crucial to an understanding of the mechanics of lowest-low fertility (Kohler et al. 2002) in Japan.

4.3 Social Background of Fertility Change

As discussed in Chap. 2, human actions are taken within the context of a human society, and one's choice of actions is affected by the social structure in which one is involved. Since fertility behaviour is one of social actions, we can, of course, conclude that fertility behaviour is influenced by social factors. In this section, we will discuss the relation between social factors and fertility behaviour in Japan.

The first point to be considered in our examination of socio-economic factors is an increase in the female enrolment rate in universities and colleges (Hodge and Ogawa 1991; Retherford and Ogawa 2006; Retherford et al. 1996). As already shown in Graph 3.9, the percentage of men enrolled in 2-year junior colleges and 4-year universities increased from 29.2 % in 1970 to 57.7 % in 2010, whereas the percentage for women rose from 17.7 to 56.0 % in the same period. Hence, it follow that, over the past 40 years, the male percentage figures doubled, but for females, the percentage figures more than tripled. According to the human capital theory (Becker 1975), the earning capacity in the labour market is a positive increasing function of educational level. Hence, compared with women who terminate their education at a high school level, those who enjoy a university education will earn a higher wage. In fact, for women in the 25–29 age group within the manufacturing industry in 2010, the average monthly wage was 214,000 yen for high school graduates and 257,000 yen for university graduates (Ministry of Labour, Health and Welfare 2012).

This brings us to our second point. In tandem with a rise in the female enrolment rate in tertiary education, female labour participation rates in non-agricultural industries have also increased. For instance, the percentage of women aged 20–44 at work in non-agricultural industries rose from 46.9 % in 1970 to 65.3 % in 2010 (see Graph 3.8). This evidence indicates that more Japanese women are engaged in paid work outside the home. In addition to the expansion of employment opportunities for women, the female average monthly wage of the manufacturing industry rose from 116,900 yen in 1980 to 227,600 yen in 2010. As a result, the wage gap between men and women has narrowed, with the ratio of women's over men's monthly average wage rising from 0.59 in 1980 to 0.71 in 2010 (Ministry of Labour, Health and Welfare 2012).

As discussed in detail in Chap. 2, an increase in women's earning capacity seems to have a negative effect on women's fertility in Japan. More specifically, according to New Home Economics theory, fertility is negatively related to the opportunity cost of rearing children (Butz and Ward 1979; Mincer 1963). Since, assuming traditional gender roles, much of a mother's time is spent bearing children and caring for infants and children, paid employment and childbearing are mutually exclusive for most women, at least for a few years. Where women have little opportunity for high-salaried employment, their earnings lost through bearing children and caring for them will be low. However, where women's opportunity for highly paid work increases, the opportunity cost (=forgone wages) imposed on women who bear and care for children will become higher. In fact, Osawa (1988) observed in Japan that a wife's educational qualifications had a negative relation to the number of children ever-born.

Furthermore, we may notice that, owing to a low level of governmental support for working mothers, making work and childrearing compatible is quite difficult for women in Japan (Gauthier 1996). For instance, Japanese parents can take parental leave until their child celebrates its first birthday, while a parental leave of 480 days is given to Swedish parents. In addition, the percentage of pay received during this period was 50 % in the Japan, whereas it reached fully 74 % in Sweden (Fukuda 2003a, b). Furthermore, as gender equality in the household is comparatively rare in Japan, women tend to perform much more housework than men. In fact, the average time spent per week on domestic work and childcare was 23 min for employed husbands aged 30 through 44, compared to 241 min for employed wives (Ministry of Internal Affairs and Communications 2012). Under these conditions, it is likely that married women in Japan will choose to have fewer children to avoid a loss of wages and to reconcile the conflict between employment and childrearing (Brodmann et al. 2007; Hochschild and Machung 2003).

It should, however, be borne in mind that the causal relation between fertility behaviour and women's employment may be more complicated than expected. On one hand, as more women are oriented towards employment or a career, rather than motherhood, they may have fewer children. On the other hand, a reduction in family size may allow more women to be engaged in paid employment (Jones 1981; Weller 1977). In the first case, labour force participation affects family size; in the second case, family size affects labour force participation. Thus, much caution is required to determine the causal link between fertility and women's employment.

In addition, we need to point out that the standards of excellence which parents set for their children have risen in Japan (Hashimoto 1974, 1980; Yamamura 1975). As mentioned earlier, Japan is seeing an upward trend in its percentage of men and women attending junior colleges and universities. From this evidence, we may infer that Japanese parents want their children to become what may be called children of higher quality. As discussed in Chap. 2, this situation may reduce the demand for children, for a household's income has an interactive relation between the quantity and quality of children (Becker and Lewis 1973).

Although the economic theory of fertility presents a plausible explanation with regard to the relation between recent economic circumstances and fertility behaviour in Japan, it is debatable whether Japanese fertility patterns are entirely attributable to economic factors. As seen in Chap. 2, the ideational theory claims that the weakening of traditional values and the spread of individualistic attitudes, following the satisfaction of material needs, are important factors in causing a change in fertility behaviour in European countries. If this theory is able to account for childbearing patterns in developed countries, it may be that Japanese fertility behaviour also takes root in these ideational changes. As argued in the previous chapter, Japan has experienced similar attitudinal changes. More specifically, the percentage of Japanese women seeking an individualistic lifestyle has increased over the past few decades. A growing number of people prefer to pursue their self-fulfilment and own goals instead of getting married and becoming a parent (see Graph 3.10). This evidence indicates that individualistic attitudes have spread among Japanese people. Similarly, the conventional Japanese inter-generational relationship has weakened and no longer holds the overwhelming influence that it once held. Japanese people tend to depend less on their children for their livelihood in old age (see Graph 3.11). The attenuation of these traditional values might lead to a decision to remain childless.

For further evidence of individualistic attitudes among Japanese people, we will look at the results of the national opinion survey conducted by the Cabinet Office in 2008 (Cabinet Office 2009). Graph 4.5 displays the difficulties involved in the rearing of children. Admittedly, the cost of education produced the highest percentage with regard to difficulty in the rearing of children (=45.8 %), with the financial burden involved in childrearing yielding the second highest figure (=25.5 %). The evidence indicates that maintaining or enhancing the quality of children is a primary concern in rearing children. However, a number of individualistic reasons comprised a considerable percentage among the categories, which

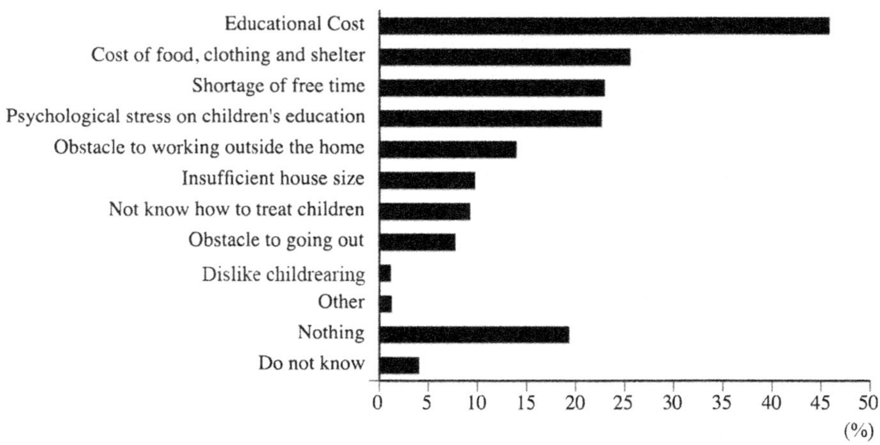

Graph 4.5 Difficulty in rearing children (multiple-choice question). *Note* The total number of respondents was 5494 (men and women over age 20). *Source* Cabinet Office (2009). National Opinion Survey on Social Life

suggests that many Japanese people place much importance on pursuing their own lifestyle. To take a case in point, respondents who thought that childrearing would shorten their amount of free time numbered 22.9 %, commanding the third highest percentage.

In addition to this, there is the question of whether children may be regarded as simple consumer goods. Clearly, a most important assumption in New Home Economics theory is that, in developed countries, having children is identical to consuming other consumer goods in respect of bringing satisfaction to parents (Blake 1967, 1968; Becker 1981; Willis 1973, 1987). However, this assumption may not entirely hold for Japanese parents; having children is endowed with meaning for them in a variety of ways. As far as Graph 4.6 shows, the percentage of respondents to a 2008 National Opinion Survey who agreed that one of the benefits of rearing children was "bringing happiness" stood at 43.5 %, which may perhaps indicate that these respondents think of children as consumable goods. However, the "help me mature as a person" benefit reached fully 53.0 % among respondents. Furthermore, the "strengthening of family ties" benefit commanded a 57.8 % response, with the chance to see a child mature as a person topping the list. This evidence suggests that the motivations behind Japanese fertility behaviour are far more complex and compelling than a simple perception of children as consumer goods.

In view of the above discussion, we can say that his relation between economic and ideational factors and current Japanese fertility behaviour are richly nuanced and complex. Admittedly, Japanese socio-economic conditions have indeed rendered the having of children more costly. However, at the same time, the attitudes of Japanese people have also changed in such a way as to emphasize the autonomy of the individual. Therefore, we need to examine Japanese fertility behaviour from economic and attitudinal aspects.

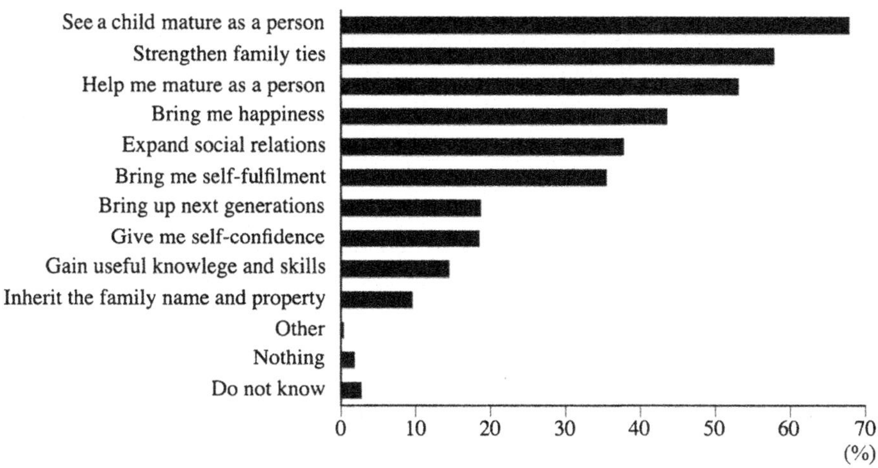

Graph 4.6 Benefits of rearing children (multiple-choice question). *Note* The total number of respondents was 5494 (men and women over age 20). *Source* Cabinet Office (2009). National Opinion Survey on Social Life

4.4 Data, Method and Variables for the Analysis of Fertility Behaviour

As mentioned in Chap. 2, a couple of analytical frameworks have already been presented for fertility behaviour (Andorka 1978; Becker 1960, 1976; Bulatao and Lee 1983; Caldwell 1982, 2006; Davis and Blake 1956; Easterlin 1978; Friedlander and Silver 1967). Referring to these frameworks, we shall describe data, method and variables employed in our analysis.

The present analysis, like the case of Chap. 3, uses data from the Japanese Generations and Gender Survey (JGGS). This is a nationwide panel survey and was conducted in 2004 for the first time. Thereafter, its follow-up surveys were carried out in 2007 and 2010. Taking reproductive span into consideration, we analysed married men and women who were under age 45 at the time of the first survey. As seen in Graph 4.3, since almost all children are born within wedlock in Japan, we excluded respondents who did not get married at the time of the first survey. Moreover, since the JGGS does not have sufficient information on the childbearing history of respondents who have experienced a divorce or separation through the death of a spouse, these respondents were also excluded from the analysis. As a result, 532 men and 842 women were used for this analysis. Since we examine the probability of additional childbirth after the first wave of the JGGP, the dependent variable of our analytical model is the hazard rate of respondents' having an additional child after the year 2004.

As in the case of marriage behaviour in Chap. 3, we employ the latent class event-history analysis in the present study (Hagenaars 1993; Hagenaars and McCutcheon 2002; Vermunt 1997). Since details of the latent class analysis were already explained in the preceding chapter, we do not dwell on this statistical method here. Moreover, like the case of Chap. 3, propensity score weighting is used in this analysis to exclude a bias caused by sample attrition (Guo and Fraser 2014). More specifically, the probability of a respondent's remaining in the sample was first estimated by logistic regression[2]. Then, an inverse of the estimated probability is used as a value of sample weight.

4.4.1 Socio-economic Variables

We shall examine the effects of three socio-economic variables on fertility behaviour: the husband's annual income, the wife's annual income and the wife's employment status.

---

[2]The propensity scores were calculated by the following logistic regression.

$$\log\left(\frac{q}{1-q}\right) = \alpha + \beta_1(\text{sex}) + \beta_2(\text{age}) + \beta_3(\text{marital status})$$
$$+ \beta_4(\text{the years of living in your current house})$$
$$+ \beta_5(\text{educational attainment}) + \beta_6(\text{residential prefecture})$$
$$+ \beta_7(\text{the number of childrenever} - \text{born})$$

Here, q is the probability of respondents' remaining in our sample

In this analysis, the husband's annual income was divided into three categories: (1) less than 4,000,000 yen; (2) 4,000,000–7,990,000 yen; and (3) equal or more than 8,000,000 yen. Several demographic studies have investigated the influence of the husband's income on fertility behaviour, especially relating to economic development in less developed countries. In most cases, a more or less positive link between fertility and income was found in the results of multiple regression analyses employing territorial cross-sectional and time-series data. Likewise, recent macro-level studies of industrialized countries also reveal a positive relation between fertility and a husband's income, which indicates that a higher income leads to higher fertility (Ahn and Mira 2001; Butz and Ward 1979; Ermisch 1970, 1979; Wilkinson 1973). If children can be regarded as consumer goods, these results suggest that a husband's higher income will increase the motivation to have more children. As mentioned before, however, it is likely that there is the interactive relation between the quantity and quality of children in Japan. If there is a strong tendency for enhancing the quality of children, a higher husband's income will lead to having fewer high-quality children.

The wife's annual income is categorized into four groups: (1) no income; (2) less than 1,000,000 yen; (3) 1,000,000–2,990,000 yen; and (4) equal or more than 3,000,000 yen. For women engaged in paid work outside the home, their income can be regarded as an index of her opportunity cost, assuming a traditional gender role. Hence, the opportunity cost of bearing and rearing children rises in tandem with an increase in the wife's annual income. As argued in the previous section, since women's income is on the increase in Japan, this variable is more likely to have a negative effect on fertility behaviour.

We classified the wife's employment status into three types: (1) not working, (2) part-time worker and (3) full-time worker. As seen in the previous section, the women's labour force participation rate is considerably high in contemporary Japan. As rearing infants and children is a time-intensive activity, working and childbearing are mutually exclusive for most women, at least for a few years. This situation may force them to be faced with a choice between continuing to work and interrupting employment. Thus, it is assumed that women in full-time employment should, *ceteris paribus*, have fewer children. However, this is not always the case in the relationship between fertility and woman's employment. Some studies indicate that the relationship between the two factors has changed in developed countries (Engelhardt et al. 2004; Engelhardt and Prskawetz 2004; Kögel 2004). More specifically, the women's labour force participation rate was negatively correlated with the TPFR in OECE countries before the mid-1980s, but thereafter, the former rate was positively connected to the latter rate. In fact, the level of fertility is high for mothers employed outside the home in Norway and Sweden (Hoem and Hoem 1989; Hoem 1993; Kravdal 1992). For instance, the labour force participation rate for Swedish women with at least one child aged 0–6 was 85.4 % in 1991. However, owing to a low level of governmental support for working mothers, it may be very difficult for women to make employment and childrearing compatible in Japan (Fukuda 2003a, b). In short, the relation between women's employment and fertility behaviour is considerably affected by the social conditions surrounding employees. With a relatively less family-friendly situation in mind, Japanese women in full employment are likely to have a lower probability of having an additional child.

4.4.2 Ideational and Attitudinal Variables

Since the JGGS had questions to ask about respondents' views concerning marriage, children and family, they were used to examine the effects of ideational factors on fertility behaviour. We used the following six opinion items for our analysis:

1. It is the eldest son's duty to look after his parents.
2. The main purpose of marriage is to have children.
3. It is acceptable for a man and woman to live together without being married.
4. It is acceptable for a couple with an unhappy marriage to get a divorce, even if they have children.
5. A man can have a full and satisfying life without marrying (only for men),
6. A woman can have a full and satisfying life without marrying (only for women).

Five answering categories were provided for each statement in the questionnaire: (1) Strongly agree, (2) Agree, (3) Uncertain, (4) Disagree and (5) Strongly disagree. For each opinion item, respondents were asked to choose the single answering category closest to their view at the time of the survey. For the sake of convenience, if a respondent chose "Strongly agree" or "Agree", we combined them into the "Agree" group in this analysis. Likewise, responses of "Disagree" or "Strongly disagree" both fell into the "Disagree" category. We will examine the influence of attitudes on fertility behaviour by using these categorical variables.

4.4.3 Control Variables

Six variables were employed as control variables in the analysis. The first control variable is the husband's participation of domestic work. Admittedly, it is difficult for parents to reconcile employment outside the home and childrearing. However, to what extent these two activities are compatible depends on the way domestic burdens are shared between a husband and wife. In other words, opportunities for paid work are affected by the structures of constraint (Joshi 1998). Where domestic tasks are shared equally between a father and mother, it will be, *ceteris paribus*, easier for the mother to work outside family. In contrast, where childcare and household chores are exclusively imposed on a mother, it is likely to be quite difficult for her to be engaged in gainful employment outside the home. Thus, the active participation of the father in housework will reduce the influence of women's employment on fertility behaviour. It is, therefore, necessary to control the level of a husband's participation in domestic work when examining the influence of a wife's employment on fertility behaviour.

A husband's domestic work score was used as an indicator of his involvement in housework. The JGGS questionnaire contains questions referring to a husband's involvement in housework. The degree of involvement in housework was measured in terms of four domestic chores: (1) cooking and cleaning after meals; (2) doing laundry; (3) cleaning house; and (4) grocery shopping. A respondent chose one out of six answers regarding the frequency of her and her partner's participation in each domestic chore: (1) almost everyday; (2) three or four times a week; (3) one or two times a week; (4) one to three times a month; (5) seldom; or (6) not at all. Based on the answers to these questions, we constructed a score that indicates the level of a husband's involvement in housework. More specifically, if a husband participated in each item of housework most frequently, a score of 6 was given. In contrast, where he did no domestic work at all, his involvement was valued at 1. Subsequently, we summed up the values a husband earned for these questions. This was termed a "husband's domestic work score". Since Cronbach's coefficient alpha of this score reached 0.77 for the first wave, 0.79 for the second wave and 0.75 for the third wave, this score has a sufficient degree of reliability and consistency. According to the husband's domestic work score, the level of his housework was divided into three: (1) high, (2) medium and (3) low. The "high" group was made up of husbands whose scores stood higher than one-third from the top. Husbands whose scores fell between one-third and two-thirds from the top belonged to the "medium" group. The "low" group was comprised of husbands whose scores were below one-third from the bottom.

The second control variable is a respondent's type of natal residential area, as it has been pointed out that this affects fertility patterns. For instance, Easterlin (1971) finds that a married couple brought up in an urban area is likely to have fewer children than a married couple brought up in a rural area. In this analysis, a respondent's type of natal residential area was used a control variable. In sociological literature, it is stated that social norms are internalized through the process of socialization in childhood. It is thus possible for a person who grew up in a rural area to be engaged in more traditional norms than an otherwise similar person who grew up in an urban area. As this difference in location of upbringing may affect childbearing behaviour, a respondent's natal residential area was employed as a control variable.

In addition, four demographic covariates were used as control variables: the number of children ever-born; the birth cohort; the marriage age; and the duration of marriage. As mentioned earlier, the dependent variable of this analysis is the hazard rate of having an additional child. When contraception is widely practised, a decision on whether to bear an additional child depends on the number of children a couple have ever had. In particular, when a couple have a target number of children they wish to have, this factor plays a critical role in their fertility behaviour.

Respondents' birth cohort is also an important control factor. People born in the same time frame will share common experiences in life and may take a similar life course (Ryder 1965). For instance, children who underwent the great depression tended to be economically independent at an earlier stage of their lives (Elder 1977). In short, since birth cohort itself may have an impact on demographic behaviour, it is necessary to control the influence of this factor.

Moreover, assuming that the frequency of coitus and abortions, and the level of birth control are constant, the risk of having children depends on marriage age and the duration of marriage. More specifically, a biological risk of conception increases when the age at marriage is lower and the marriage lasts longer. Thus, we included these variables in our analytical model.

4.5 Descriptive Analysis of Fertility Patterns

Before exploring Japanese fertility behaviour by latent class event-history analysis, we will, in this section, show the results of descriptive analyses derived from our survey data. Since our data are obtained from panel surveys, exploratory variables may change their values from one wave to another. Yet, the main focus of this section is to give an overall picture of the relation between key exploratory variables and bearing an additional child. Thus, we, in Sect. 4.4, concentrate on values of exploratory variables at the first wave of the panel survey.

Table 4.1 displays the percentage of respondents who had an additional child from the first wave to the third wave of the JGGS. As might be expected, the percentage of additional birth was low at a relative higher-order birth (see Table 4.1). The percentage of parents who had additional children was only 3.9 % when they already had three children at the time of the first survey. Similarly, the figure stood at 7.3 % for parents who had equal to or more than four children. In contrast, the percentage experiencing additional childbirth was 50.0 % for childless respondents and 43.0 % for parents with one child. Since the percentage of having an additional child is great for these parity groups, we can argue that the two-child norm is still alive in Japanese society.

Table 4.1 The number of children ever-born and additional birth (%)

Number of children (at wave 1)	Having an additional child		
	No	Yes	*N*
0	50.0	50.0	106
1	57.0	43.0	258
2	88.8	11.2	543
3	96.1	3.9	256
4 or more	92.7	7.3	42
N	966	238	1204

Source The Japanese generations and gender survey

Concerning a husband's annual income, a lower husband's income leads to a greater percentage of having additional children (see Panel (a) of Table 4.2). About 30 % of husbands who earned less than 4,000,000 yen per year had a child, while the percentage fell to 13.5 % for those who earned equal or more than 8,000,000 yen. This finding should, however, be taken with reservations, for the amount of annual income tends to be smaller when a husband is younger. To control this age effect, Panel (b) of Table 4.2 displays the relation between annual income and childbirth for husbands in their 30s. Interestingly, the negative relation between income level and the percentage of having an additional child as seen in Panel (a) weakens in Panel (b). The percentages are almost equal regardless of the husbands' income. The evidence indicates that a husband's income has no clear bearing on fertility behaviour when he is relatively young.

No salient difference in the percentage of bearing an additional child is identified for wives' income (see Table 4.3). Although the no-income category yields a high percentage of bearing an additional child, the remaining income groups do not show a clear difference in the percentage. The experience rate of additional childbirth in the three categories stood at around 16 %, regardless of the level of wives' annual income. It is therefore quite likely that the women's opportunity cost of bearing and rearing children has a clear impact on fertility behaviour.

Table 4.2 Husband's annual income and additional birth (%)

Husband's income (at wave 1)	Having an additional child		
	No	Yes	*N*
(a) All husbands			
−3,990,000 yen	72.5	27.5	404
4,000,000–7,990,000 yen	83.7	16.3	674
8,000,000 yen	86.5	13.5	126
N	966	238	1204
(b) Husbands in their 30s			
−3,990,000 yen	70.8	29.2	216
4,000,000–7,990,000 yen	77.4	22.6	385
8,000,000 yen	77.6	22.4	58
N	496	163	659

Source The Japanese generations and gender survey

Table 4.3 Wife's annual income and additional birth (%)

Wife's income (at wave 1)	Having an additional child		
	No	Yes	*N*
None	75.9	24.1	489
−990,000 yen	84.3	15.7	318
1,000,000–2,990,000 yen	82.2	17.8	247
3,000,000 yen	82.7	17.3	150
N	966	238	1204

Source The Japanese generations and gender survey

As far as Table 4.4 shows, women's employment outside the home tends to deter childbirth. The percentage of experiencing an additional birth was 13.6 % for wives in full-time work and 12.0 % for those in part-time work, while fully 28.6 % of wives not in employment bore a child during the period between the first wave and the third wave of the survey (see Panel (a) of Table 4.4). Interestingly, the relation between the two variables changed considerably when we controlled the level of a husband's housework participation. For instance, when a husband rarely did domestic work, only five per cent of full-time wives gave birth (see Panel (b) of Table 4.4). In contrast, when the level of husbands' participation in domestic work was high, full-time working wives who bore an additional child reached 11 % (see Panel (c) of Table 4.4). We can, therefore, argue that the relation between women's employment and fertility behaviour depends on men's participation in domestic work.

Let us turn to the influence of ideational factors on fertility behaviour. Table 4.5 displays the relation between respondents' attitudes and additional childbearing. First of all, regarding Item (a) of Table 4.5, both men and women do not have a clear relation between the two variables. The percentage of having an additional child did not vary whether or not respondents upheld traditional filial duties. Second, a consistent relation was clearly observed between Items (c), (e) and (f) of Table 4.5. For instance, 28.5 % of husbands who agreed with Item (c) had an additional child, whereas the percentage fell to 18.3 % for those who disagreed with

Table 4.4 Wife's employment status and additional birth (%)

Wife's employment status (at wave 1)	Having an additional child		
	No	Yes	*N*
(a) All husband			
Not working	71.4	28.6	511
Part-time	86.4	13.6	568
Full-time	88.0	12.0	125
N	966	238	1204
(b) Low participation husbands			
Not Working	72.9	27.1	133.0
Part-time	89.1	10.9	156.0
Full-time	94.9	5.1	39.0
N	273	55	328
(c) High participation husbands			
Not working	66.7	33.3	138
Part-time	85.4	14.6	205
Full-time	88.9	11.1	36
N	299	80.0	379

The high participation group was made up of husbands whose domestic work scores stood higher than one-third from the top. The low participation group was comprised of husbands whose domestic work scores were below one-third from the bottom
Source The Japanese generations and gender survey

Table 4.5 Value-orientations and additional birth (%)

Men (at wave 1) (at wave 1)	Having an additional child			Women (at wave 1)	Having an additional child		
	No	Yes	*N*		No	Yes	*N*
(a) It is the eldest son's duty to look after his parents							
Agree	74.5	25.5	204	Agree	83.2	16.8	161
Uncertain	78.1	21.9	219	Uncertain	81.7	18.3	393
Disagree	76.0	24.0	50	Disagree	84.8	15.3	177
N	361	112	473	*N*	605	126	731
(b) The main purpose of marriage is to have children							
Agree	80.5	19.5	123	Agree	83.4	16.6	151
Uncertain	75.3	24.7	235	Uncertain	82.5	17.6	359
Disagree	73.9	26.1	115	Disagree	82.8	17.2	221
N	361	112	473	*N*	605	126	731
(c) It is acceptable for a man and woman to live together without being married							
Agree	71.5	28.5	228	Agree	79.0	21.0	348
Uncertain	80.3	19.7	152	Uncertain	85.8	14.2	233
Disagree	81.7	18.3	93	Disagree	86.7	13.3	150
N	361	112	473	*N*	605	126	731
(d) It is acceptable for a couple with an unhappy marriage to get a divorce, even if they have children							
Agree	76.4	23.6	250	Agree	82.4	17.6	558
Uncertain	75.2	24.8	145	Uncertain	83.0	17.1	129
Disagree	78.2	21.8	78	Disagree	86.4	13.6	44
N	361	112	473	*N*	605	126	731
(e) A man can have a full and satisfying life without marrying				*(f) A woman can have a full and satisfying life without marrying*			
Agree	79.2	20.8	120	Agree	84.4	15.6	231
Uncertain	76.9	23.1	242	Uncertain	83.8	16.2	394
Disagree	72.1	27.9	111	Disagree	75.5	24.5	106
N	361	112	473	*N*	605	126	731

Source The Japanese generations and gender survey

Item (c). In the same vein, the percentage of bearing a child reached 24.1 % for wives who agreed with Item (c) of Table 4.5, compared with 13.3 % for those who disagreed with the statement. These findings indicate that respondents with conventional attitudes towards marriage have a greater risk of bearing an additional child. Third, Item (b) of Table 4.5 shows a clear difference in the relation between the attitudinal and demographic variables for only men. More specifically, of male respondents who thought that the main purpose of marriage is to have children, 19.5 % had a child, while the figure reached 26.1 % for those who disagreed with the item. Yet, such a feature was not identified for female respondents. Fourth, the percentage of bearing a child differs between the answering categories of Item (d) for women only. Wives who had an additional child stood at 17.6 % of those who agreed with the divorce of a couple with children, whereas 13.6 % of women who disagreed with it bore a child. Since Item (d) measures the extent to which children are important in one's life in comparison with oneself, more child-centred women tended to have children.

Since the descriptive bivariate analysis which we carried out in this section shows only a covariant relation between the two variables, it is almost impossible to draw a definite conclusion regarding the effects of economic and ideational factors on fertility patterns. Hence, we will, in the following sections, conduct the latent class event-history analysis in order to examine the effects of the two factors on fertility behaviour in more detail.

4.6 Finding Latent Classes for Fertility Behaviour

In the previous section, we looked at the relation between ideational factors and fertility behaviour. Yet, since respondent's attitudes are measured by multiple items, understanding the overall relation between attitudes and fertility behaviour is not straightforward. Taking this point into consideration, we will, in this section, classify attitudes into a few groups by using latent class analysis.

Table 4.6 displays the model evaluation of latent class analysis. With regard to husbands, the chi-square test is statistically significant for the Class 2 model, indicating that it is considerably different from an unconstrained model. Thus, the Class 2 model lacks sufficient goodness of fit. On the other hand, since the Class 3 and Class 4 models yield insignificance in the chi-square test, they are not different from the null model and have sufficient goodness of fit. Yet, the value of BIC (Bayesian Information Criterion) is smaller for the Class 3 model than the Class 4 model. Since a smaller BIC value means a better fit of a model (Raftery 1995), we can argue that the Class 3 model is most parsimonious and appropriate for a classification of husbands' latent class. Wives also turned out a similar result to

Table 4.6 Model evaluation of latent class analysis

Number of latent class	Degrees of freedom	Log-likelihood	Chi-square p value	BIC	*N*
Husbands					
2	103	−2337.90	0.00	4805.14	473
3	92	−2301.08	0.09	4799.24	473
4	81	−2276.41	0.14	4817.66	473
Wives					
2	221	−3394.84	0.00	6928.16	731
3	210	−3362.52	0.10	6936.06	731
4	199	−3341.53	0.25	6966.61	731

Source The Japanese generations and gender survey

husbands in model fitness. The chi-square test is significant for the female Class 2 model, making its goodness of fit insufficient. Although the Class 3 and Class 4 models show sufficient goodness of fit by chi-square test, the value of BIC is smaller for the former model than the latter model. Thus, Class 3 is best fitted to wives. In conclusion, it follows that respondents' attitudes are classified into three latent classes for both husbands and wives.

Table 4.7 displays the relation between the latent classes and the conditional probability of each item. First of all, let us look at features of husbands' latent classes. Items (3) and (4) yield a high probability for the "Agree" category in Class 1. For example, the probability of agreeing that it is acceptable for a man and woman to live together without being married reached 0.64. In contrast,

Table 4.7 Latent class and conditional probability

Husbands				Wives			
	Class 1	Class 2	Class 3		Class 1	Class 2	Class 3
Item (1)				Item (1)			
Agree	0.26	0.25	0.63	Agree	0.18	0.23	0.31
Uncertain	0.41	0.74	0.34	Uncertain	0.54	0.58	0.47
Disagree	0.33	0.01	0.03	Disagree	0.28	0.19	0.23
Item (2)				Item (2)			
Agree	0.06	0.03	0.51	Agree	0.16	0.10	0.46
Uncertain	0.11	0.95	0.48	Uncertain	0.41	0.71	0.35
Disagree	0.83	0.02	0.02	Disagree	0.43	0.19	0.18
Item (3)				Item (3)			
Agree	0.64	0.49	0.39	Agree	0.71	0.28	0.25
Uncertain	0.22	0.41	0.34	Uncertain	0.18	0.59	0.23
Disagree	0.15	0.10	0.28	Disagree	0.11	0.13	0.52
Item (4)				Items (4)			
Agree	0.62	0.57	0.46	Agree	0.91	0.66	0.58
Uncertain	0.20	0.42	0.31	Uncertain	0.07	0.32	0.20
Disagree	0.19	0.01	0.24	Disagree	0.02	0.02	0.22
Item (5)				Item (6)			
Agree	0.37	0.23	0.19	Agree	0.56	0.16	0.01
Uncertain	0.37	0.75	0.46	Uncertain	0.42	0.80	0.43
Disagree	0.26	0.02	0.34	Disagree	0.02	0.04	0.56
Overall class size	0.27	0.26	0.47	Overall class size	0.47	0.31	0.22

Item statements are as follows:
(1) It is the eldest son's duty to look after his parents
(2) The main purpose of marriage is to have children
(3) It is acceptable for a man and woman to live together without being married
(4) It is acceptable for a couple with an unhappy marriage to get a divorce, even if they have children
(5) A man can have a full and satisfying life without marrying (only for men)
(6) A woman can have a full and satisfying life without marrying (only for women)
Source The Japanese generations and gender survey

probability of the "Disagree" category in Item (2) was quite high, standing at 0.83 in Class 1. In short, husbands in this class tend to strongly disagree that the main purpose of marriage is to have children. Since Items (3) and (4) measure the level of acceptance of untraditional and individualistic values, it follows that respondents who agree with these statements have a progressive attitude. Furthermore, as the opinion of Item (2) holds to traditional ideas on marriage, opposition to the item indicates that a respondent has a progressive attitude. Taking these results into consideration, Class 1 can be termed a "progressive" group. With reference to Class 2, the most conspicuous feature is that the "Uncertain" category bears a high proportion in all items. For example, the probability of the "Uncertain" category was 0.74 for Item (1), 0.95 for Item (2) and 0.75 for Item (5). This response pattern indicates that the respondents do not have a decisive view about the items. Thus, Class 2 can be named a "neutral" group. Class 3 yields a high probability for the "Agree" category in Items (1) and (2). The probability of agreeing with the opinion was 0.63 in Item (1) and 0.51 in Item (2). Hence, husbands in this class support the eldest son's filial duty and marriage for procreation. In contrast, as seen in Item (3) or Item (5), cohabitation and lifelong celibacy tend to be unacceptable in Class 3. This evidence indicates that Class 3 holds a strong commitment to traditional values. We can, therefore, call Class 3 a "conservative" group.

Now let us turn to the features of wives' latent classes. The probability of choosing the "Agree" category is high for Items (3), (4) and (6) in Class 1. The figure stood at 0.71 in Item (3), 0.91 in Item (4) and 0.56 in Item (6). In brief, wives in this class tend to support cohabitation, the divorce of parents with children and lifelong celibacy. By contrast, women in Class 1 tend to disagree that the main purpose of marriage is to have children. This response pattern indicates that respondents have untraditional and self-oriented attitudes towards marriage and family. Class 1 can therefore be called a "progressive" group. In Class 2, wives, as a whole, tend to choose the "Uncertain" with a high probability. In fact, the probability of falling into this category reached 0.71 in Item (2) and 0.80 in Item (6). The remaining items also show a relatively high probability of belonging to the "Uncertain" category. Judging from this response pattern, Class 2 can be classified into a "neutral" group. Class 3, in contrast to Class 1, has a response pattern in favour of traditional values on marriage and family. While the probability of choosing the "Agree" category is high for Item (2), Item (6) yields a large probability for the "Disagree" category. In other words, wives who belong to Class 1 tend to support marriage for the sake of procreation and to oppose a lifelong celibacy strongly. As far as these features show, we may term this class a "conservative" group.

Interestingly, there is a gender difference in the overall size of latent classes. The conservative group is largest for men, commanding 47 % of all husbands. In contrast, the progressive group is the greatest latent class, containing 47 % of the female respondents. Thus, we can argue that Japanese husbands are more conservative than wives in terms of attitudes towards marriage and family.

4.7 Results of the Latent Class Event-History Analysis of Childbirth

The results of latent class event-history analysis for husbands are displayed in Table 4.8. Model 1 of Table 4.8 includes only demographic control variables as covariates. This model gives the first impression that the duration of marriage has a strong influence on the hazard of having an additional child. There is a high probability of childbirths occurring within the first six years of marriage, but thereafter they cease to happen gradually. In contrast, a husband's age at marriage hardly affects the hazard rate. None of the coefficients for this variable are statistically significant. It thus follows that the timing of men's entering marriage hardly plays a role in determining fertility patterns. Likewise, the birth cohort also yields no statistically significant coefficient, indicating that the pattern of childbirth does not differ between birth cohorts. Interestingly, the "Childless" category in the number of children ever-born shows a significant positive coefficient, while the coefficient for the "2 Children or More" category is not significant. This result suggests that, since childlessness is unpopular in Japan, a risk of having children is relatively great for married men without children. In fact, the 14th Japanese Fertility Survey finds that only 4.2 % of married couples planned to remain childless (National Institute of Population and Social Security Research 2012).

Models 2 and 3 in Table 4.8 were carried out to examine the influence of couples' incomes on fertility behaviour. No significant effect was observed with regard to husbands' incomes. Similarly, the levels of wives' income showed no significant coefficient, although only the "no income" category turned out a significantly high hazard rate. As seen earlier in Table 4.3, most Japanese people feel that bringing up children is financially burdensome. Despite this fact, a lower income does not always lead to a smaller probability of childbirth. It is, therefore, safe to say that the cost of rearing children does not, in reality, affect Japanese fertility behaviour. Rather, the wife's employment status plays a crucial role in whether a couple have children (see Table 4.8, Model 4). Compared with wives who were not in employment, those who worked part-time turned out to have about a 60 % lower hazard rate of having a child. Similarly, the hazard rate was approximately 70 % lower for wives in full-time employment. Furthermore, the BIC value was smaller for Model 4 than for Model 3 in Table 4.8, which means that the former model has a better goodness of fit than the latter model. We can therefore argue that wives' employment status strongly affects fertility behaviour in Japan. Interestingly, the level of a husband's participation in domestic work does not affect the hazard rate significantly (see Table 4.8, Model 5). This evidence may indicate that the amount of housework done by a husband is not sufficient for reconciling the conflict between wives' employment and domestic work. Here, suffice it to say that the extent of a husband's participation in domestic work exerts no substantial influence on fertility behaviour.

With regard to the impact of ideational factors on fertility behaviour, Model 6 of Table 4.8 shows that more progressive attitudes lead to a significantly lower risk

Table 4.8 Results of latent class event-history analysis for husbands

	Model 1	Model 2	Model 3	Model 4	Model 5	Model 6	Model 7
Covariate	Coefficient	Coefficient	Coefficient	Coefficient	Coefficient	Coefficient	Coefficient
Constant	−2.61***	−2.55	−2.98***	6.7**	8.7**	−1.55	−0.65**
Duration of marriage+							
Less than 3 years	2.90***	2.89***	2.66***	2.60***	2.51***	3.94***	4.08***
4–6 years	2.16***	2.16***	−2.01***	2.00***	1.98 ***	3.58***	3.07***
7–9 years	1.39***	1.39***	1.32***	1.29***	2.8***	1.45	1.90***
(10–12 years)							
13–15 years	−0.90	−0.90	−0.71	−0.65	−0.63	−0.24	−2.28
16 years–	−1.82	−1.81	−1.49	−1.45	−1.39	−0.70	−3.47
Natal residential area							
(Rural)							
Urban	−0.24	−0.24	−0.28	−0.27	−0.27	−0.57	−0.86
Birth cohort							
Before 1959	−4.03	−4.21	−4.64	−4.47	−4.53	−5.16	−7.74
(1960–1964)							
1965–1969	0.36	0.37	0.47	0.48	0.56	1.53	1.10
1970–1974	0.72	0.71	0.93	0.85	0.93	2.58	1.24
After 1975	0.41	0.40	0.72	0.58	0.68	1.94	0.65
The number of children ever-born+							
Childless	0.90**	0.9**	0.83	0.71*	0.71*	1.27*	0.55*
(1 child)							
2 children or more	−0.17	−0.17	−0.59	−0.25	−0.20	−0.08	−0.61
Age at marriage							
(Under 23)							
24–26	0.58	0.60	0.66	0.61	0.60	0.62	0.32
27–29	0.93	0.95	1.09	1.00	0.96	1.73	1.24
30–32	0.57	0.58	0.73	0.61	0.64	1.93	0.78
33–35	0.94	0.96	1.24	1.06	1.11	2.98	2.99
Over 36	0.49	0.50	0.77	0.54	0.66	1.99	1.47
Husband's income+							
(Less than 4,000,000 yen)							
4,000,000–7,990,000 yen		−0.10	−0.22	−0.26	−0.28	−0.68	−0.09
8,000,000 yen		−0.13	−0.15	−0.21	−0.20	−0.06	−0.10
Wife's income+							
No income			0.54*				
(Less than 1,000,000 yen)							
1,000,000-2,990,000 yen			−0.39				
3,000,000 yen			−0.01				

(continued)

Table 4.8 (continued)

	Model 1	Model 2	Model 3	Model 4	Model 5	Model 6	Model 7
Covariate	Coefficient	Coefficient	Coefficient	Coefficient	Coefficient	Coefficient	Coefficient
Wife's employment status+							
(Not working)							
Part-time worker				−1.05**	−1.08***	−1.82***	-2.43***
Full-time worker				−1.08***	−1.14**	−2.06**	−1.89**
Husband's domestic work+							
Low					−0.32		
(Medium)							
High					0.13		
Latent class+							
(Conservative)							
Progressive						−2.39***	
Neutral						−1.77***	
Interaction term+							
(Not working* conservative)							
Part-time* conservative							5.79
Full-time* conservative							−3.09
Not working* progressive							−3.82*
Part-time* progressive							−0.11
Full-time* progressive							0.41
Not working* neutral							−2.67*
Part-time* neutral							4.52
Full-time* neutral							3.60
Log-likelihood	−208.49	−208.39	−204.77	−200.29	−199.30	−183.88	−181.40
BIC	530.36	542.75	554.42	539.15	549.78	632.31	665.13
N	473	473	473	473	473	473	473

Parentheses are reference categories
+ is a time-varying variable
Time-varying variables take values prior to the occurrence of an event
Source The Japanese generations and gender survey
$*p < 0.10$; $**p < 0.05$; $***p < 0.01$

of having an additional child. More specifically, husbands with progressive attitudes turned out to have a 90 % lower hazard rate than those with conservative attitudes. Furthermore, the hazard rate was 80 % lower even for husbands with neutral attitudes. The value of BIC is, however, smaller for Model 4 than Model 6. We can, therefore, argue that attitudinal factors exert a limited influence on fertility behaviour. Moreover, it should be noted that the impact of a husband's attitudes varies, depending on his wife's employment status (see Table 4.8, Model 7). In concrete terms, when wives are not working, their husband' attitudes have a significant effect on the probability of having a child. Yet, when wives are employed part-time or full-time, no significant influence is observed with regard to the hazard rate. In other words, a husband's attitudes do not affect fertility behaviour when his wife has economic autonomy.

Let us turn to the results of the wives' analysis. Model 1 of Table 4.9, as in Table 4.8, includes demographic control variables as covariates. The duration of marriage significantly affects the hazard rate of bearing an additional child. The hazard rate decreases as the period of marriage expands. For the wives, unlike their husbands, marriage age exerts a significant influence on the hazard rate. The risk of having an additional birth gradually increases until a wife begins to go through her 30s, and then decreases in her mid-30s. Thereafter, it rises again after age 36. It can, therefore, be argued that female marriage age plays a more important role in fertility behaviour than male marriage age. The birth cohort also affects the risk of giving birth to a child significantly. Compared with the 1960–64 birth cohort, more recent cohorts show a greater hazard rate. Thus, the risk of having children is relatively great for younger women.

Models 2 and 3 of Table 4.9 include married couples' incomes as independent variables. The husbands' incomes do not produce a significant coefficient; therefore, the level of their income does not affect the probability of giving birth to a child. Furthermore, since the coefficients of the wives' incomes are not statistically significant except for wives without income (see Table 4.9, Model 3), it follows that the direct and indirect (opportunity) costs of rearing children hardly have an influence on fertility behaviour. Rather, wives' employment status is crucial to the risk of childbearing (see Table 4.9, Model 4). Compared with wives who did not work, those in part-time employment revealed, significantly, a 65 % lower hazard rate. Likewise, the hazard rate of wives in full-time employment was approximately 40 % lower. This evidence suggests that the conflict between a family role and employment role is an obstacle to having children. Furthermore, even when the level of a husband's participation in domestic work was controlled, the wife's employment status still had a significant effect on a risk of childbirth (see Table 4.9, Model 5). Thus, the extent of a husband's participation in housework seems to have only a weak impact on harmonizing his wife's employment with her family role.

Concerning attitudinal variables, a statistically significant effect was identified in Model 6 of Table 4.9. Compared with wives who had conservative attitudes, those who held neutral attitudes yielded an 80 % lower hazard rate of having an additional child. The rate was about 90 % lower for wives with progressive attitudes. At the same time, however, the value of BIC is smaller for Model 4 than

Table 4.9 Results of latent class event-history analysis for wives

	Model 1	Model 2	Model 3	Model 4	Model 5	Model 6	Model 7
Covariate	Coefficient	Coefficient	Coefficient	Coefficient	Coefficient	Coefficient	Coefficient
Constant	−4.43	−4.35***	−4.43***	−3.68***	−3.67***	−2.64***	−2.39***
Duration of marriage+							
Less than 3 years	1.53***	1.60***	1.50***	3.4***	4.2***	7.9***	2.41***
4–6 years	0.74	0.78	0.71**	0.63*	0.67*	0.88	1.12*
7–9 years	0.41**	0.42**	0.37**	0.35**	0.37**	0.40*	0.54*
(10–12 years)							
13−15 years	−0.39	−0.38	−0.35	−0.26	−0.26	−0.17	−0.28
16 years–	−0.24	−0.23	−0.18	−0.15	−0.19	0.02	−0.10
Natal residential area							
(Rural)							
Urban	−0.02	−0.01	0.00	−0.02	−0.02	−0.07	−0.04
Birth cohort							
Before 1959	−4.74	−4.91	−4.89	−4.64	−4.77	−4.34	−4.78
(1960–1964)							
1965–1969	2.02***	2.03***	2.02***	9.9***	9.6***	2.15***	2.59***
1970–1974	2.95***	2.92***	2.94***	2.90***	2.84***	3.37***	4.25***
After 1975	3.65***	3.54***	3.56***	3 45***	3.39***	3.76***	5.24***
The number of children ever-born+							
childless	0.31*	0.32*	0.16*	0.02*	0.02*	0.14*	0.27*
(1 child)							
2 children or more	−0.15	−0.08	−0.08	−0.07	−0.10	−0.06	−0.12
Age at marriage							
(Under 23)							
24–26	0.55 *	0.59*	0.63*	0.59*	0.58*	0.59*	0.98*
27–29	1.14***	1.20***	1.23***	1.18***	1.16***	2.7***	2.13***
30–32	1.28**	1.31**	1.31**	1.17*	1.13*	1.52*	2.14*
33–35	0.61	0.56	0.61	0.60	0.50	0.50	0.14
Over 36	2.86***	2.94***	2.95***	2.82***	2.81***	3.09***	4.42***
Husband's income+							
(Less than 4,000,000 yen)							
4,000,000–7,990,000 yen		−0.42	−0.48	−0.55	−0.56	−0.54	−0.87
8,000,000 yen		−0.07	−0.15	−0.35	−0.35	−0.36	−0.35
Wife's income+							
No income			0.34**				
(Less than 1,000,000 yen)							

(continued)

Table 4.9 (continued)

	Model 1	Model 2	Model 3	Model 4	Model 5	Model 6	Model 7
Covariate	Coefficient	Coefficient	Coefficient	Coefficient	Coefficient	Coefficient	Coefficient
1,000,000–2,990,000 yen			−0.06				
3,000,000 yen			−0.06				
Wife's employment status+							
(Not working)							
Part-time worker				−1 01***	−0.99***	−1.14***	−3.10***
Full-time worker				−0.47**	−0.48**	−0.67**	−4.84***
Husband's domestic work+							
Low					−0.16		
(Medium)							
High					0.19		
Latent class+							
(Conservative)							
Progressive						−4.26*	
Neutral						−1.71***	
Interaction term+							
(Not working* conservative)							
Not working* progressive							3.25
Not working* neutral							4.11
Part-time* conservative							−0.15
Part-time* progressive							−4.67
Part-time*neutral							1.27
(Full-time* conservative)							0.15
Full-time* progressive							−4.19**
Full-time* neutral							−6.84**
Log-likelihood	−238.95	−237.54	−236.53	−230.60	−229.92	−214.94	−210.48
BIC	596.26	606.59	624.30	605.87	617.66	706.06	736.60
N	731	731	731	731	731	731	731

Parentheses are reference categories
+ is a time-varying variable
Time-varying variables take values prior to the occurrence of an event
Source the Japanese generations and gender survey
$^{*}p < 0.10$; $^{**}p < 0.05$; $^{***}p < 0.01$

Model 6. This indicates that the former model has a better goodness of fit than the latter model. Hence, although attitudinal variables affect fertility behaviour, the extent of their influence is, as a whole, not so great.

Moreover, it is worth noting that ideational factors differ in influence in accordance with a wife's employment status. More specifically, when wives are working outside the home, their attitudes significantly affect their fertility behaviour. Yet, when they work part-time, or do not work, their attitudes exert no significant influence on fertility (see Table 4.9, Model 7). It can, therefore, be seen that the influence of ideational factors is limited to women with a considerable degree of economic independence from their husbands.

4.8 An Impact of Childbirth on Attitudes

In the previous section, we examined the influence of attitudes on fertility behaviour. As discussed in Chap. 2, however, we should not ignore a reverse relation between the two factors. More specifically, it is possible that having children changes men's and women's attitudes towards partnership and family relations. In fact, it is found that the experience of independent non-family living arrangements weakens young adults' commitment to traditional family values (Waite et al. 1986). Similarly, it is pointed out that people who experienced cohabitation were more tolerant to divorce (Axinn and Thornton 1992). Taking these findings into consideration, it is necessary to investigate the impact of a life-course event on an ideational change. In this section, we investigate the influence of childbirth on attitudes.

Table 4.10 displays the association of attitudes between the first wave and the third wave of the JGGS. In our overall impression of the table, respondents' attitudes are not so stable between the two waves. The Cramer's Coefficient of Association rests at around 0.3 in most of the tables, indicating a mild connection between respondents' attitudes in the two waves of the survey. Admittedly, 70.1 % of husbands who agreed with Item (a), the eldest son's care for parents, in the first wave still stayed at the same category in the second wave. Likewise, 83.2 % of wives in the "Agree" category of Item (d), the divorce of parents with children, at the first wave remained at the same category at the second wave. We can, however, see a salient attitudinal change at Items (b), (c), (e) and (f). For an instance, while 48.8 % of wives who disagreed that the main purpose of marriage is to have children in the first wave moved to the "Uncertain" category in the third wave. Likewise, 44.2 % of husbands who agreed with Item (e), lifelong celibacy, in the first wave shifted to the "Uncertain" category in the second wave.

In order to look at an overall change in attitudes, Graph 4.7 shows a trajectory of latent classes from the first wave to the third wave of the survey. With regard to husbands, Class 1 (progressive group) decreased its size from 27 % in the first wave to 19 % in the third wave, while the size of Class 3 (conservative group) considerably fell from 47 to 23 %. In contrast, the percentage of Class 2 (neutral

Table 4.10 Value-orientations between the 1st wave and the 3rd wave

Husbands	3rd wave				Wives	3rd wave			
(a) It is the eldest son's duty to look after his parents									
1st wave	Agree	Uncertain	Disagree	*N*	1st wave	Agree	Uncertain	Disagree	*N*
Agree	70.1	25.5	4.4	204	Agree	58.4	37.3	4.4	161
Uncertain	27.4	62.1	10.5	219	Uncertain	16.0	71.0	13.0	393
Disagree	16.0	60.0	24.0	50	Disagree	5.7	49.2	45.2	177
N	211	218	44	473	*N*	167	426	138	731
Cramer's coefficient of association: 0.33					Cramer's coefficient of association: 0.40				
(b) The main purpose of marriage is to have children									
Agree	56.9	38.2	4.9	123	Agree	63.6	31.1	5.3	151
Uncertain	28.5	59.2	12.3	235	Uncertain	23.7	60.5	15.9	359
Disagree	13.9	58.3	27.8	115	Disagree	8.6	48.9	42.5	221
N	153	253	67	473	*N*	200	372	159	731
Cramer's coefficient of association: 0.27					Cramer's coefficient of association: 0.36				
(c) It is acceptable for a man and woman to live together without being married									
Agree	57.9	31.6	10.5	228	Agree	63.8	27.0	9.2	348
Uncertain	30.3	50.0	19.7	152	Uncertain	28.3	52.8	18.9	233
Disagree	7.5	38.7	53.8	93	Disagree	14.0	34.0	52.0	150
N	185	184	104	473	*N*	309	268	154	731
Cramer's coefficient of association: 0.34					Cramer's coefficient of association: 0.37				
(d) It is acceptable for a couple with an unhappy marriage to get a divorce, even if they have children									
Agree	67.2	22.4	10.4	250	Agree	83.2	15.2	1.6	558
Uncertain	41.4	40.7	17.9	145	Uncertain	52.7	39.5	7.8	129
Disagree	24.4	47.4	28.2	78	Disagree	38.6	43.2	18.2	44
N	247	152	74	473	*N*	549	155	27	731

Husbands	3rd wave			Wives	3rd wave		
Cramer's coefficient of association: 0.24				Cramer's coefficient of association: 0.26			
(e) A man can have a full and satisfying life without marrying				*(f) A woman can have a full and satisfying life without marrying*			
Agree	50.8	44.2	5.0	120	Agree	47.2	40.3	12.6	231
Uncertain	18.2	62.4	19.4	242	Uncertain	23.4	63.2	13.5	394
Disagree	13.5	40.5	46.0	111	Disagree	8.5	35.9	55.7	106
N	120	249	104	473	*N*	210	380	141	731
Cramer's coefficient of association: 0.32					Cramer's coefficient of association: 0.32				

The sum of columns in each row amounts to 100 %

Source The Japanese generations and gender survey

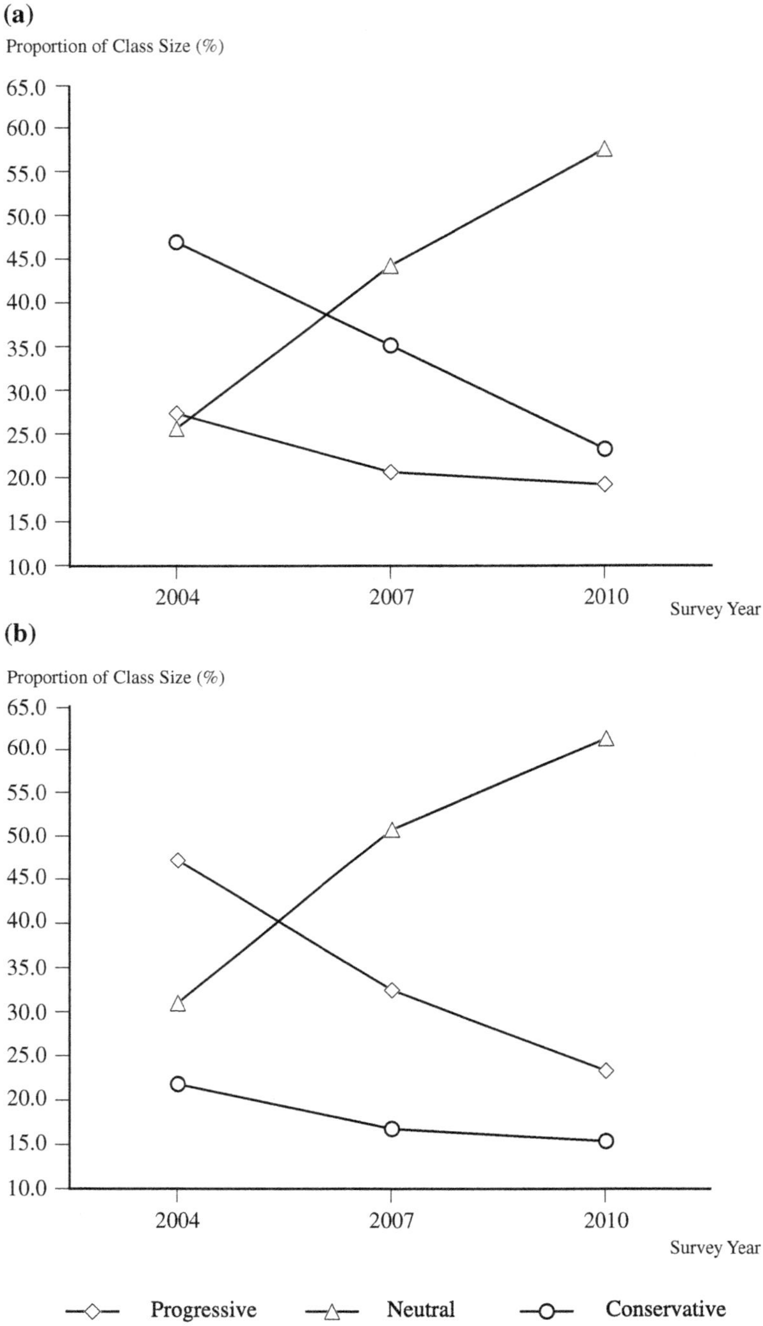

Graph 4.7 Trajectory of latent class. *Source* The Japanese generations and gender survey. **a** Husband, **b** Wife

group) rose from 27 to 58 %. Thus, it follows that, as time goes by, husband tend to have neutral attitudes to partnership and family relations. For the wives, on the other hand, Class 1 (progressive group) revealed a considerable downward trend from 47 to 23 %. By the same token, the percentage of the wives' Class 3 (conservative group) slightly fell from 22 to 15 %. In contrast, the wives' Class 2 (neutral group) drastically increased its size from 31 to 62 %. We can, therefore, argue that, like the case of husbands, wives' attitudes also become neutral with the lapse of time. In short, husbands and wives present us with similar patterns of class size change from the first to the third waves.

4.9 Results of the Logistic Latent Class Regression of Childbirth

In order to examine the influence of childbirth on attitudes, this section will present the results of logistic latent class regression (Hagenaars and McCutcheon 2002). All models employed in the analysis have random intercepts and random coefficients (for details, see Chap. 3).

Table 4.11 displays the result of the husbands' analysis. Model 1 of Table 4.11 includes demographic variables and couples' income as independent variables. First of all, demographic variables do not have a substantial influence on a husband's attitudes. In concrete terms, regression coefficients are statistically insignificant in the duration of marriage, birth cohorts, the number of children ever-born and a husband's age at marriage. This result implies that the odds ratio of the neutral over the conservative groups and the odds ratio of the progressive over the conservative group are hardly affected by demographic factors. By contrast, husbands' and wives' incomes exert salient influences on husbands' attitudes. To be concrete, compared with husbands who earned less than 4,000,000 yen a year, those who made an income of 4,000,000–7,990,000 yen reduced the odds ratios of the neutral over the conservative group by 80 % and the progressive over the conservative group by 35 %. Hence, the medium level of husbands' income leads to a conservative attitude. In contrast, when wives earned more than or equal to 3,000,000 yen a year, the odds ratio of the neutral over the conservative group was 8.7 times greater than the odds ratio for wives earning less than 1,000,000 yen per year. Similarly, the odds ratio of neutral over conservative categories rose by 9.0 times when their wives received an annual income of more than or equal to 3,000,000 yen per year. This result indicates that a greater income makes wives less conservative. Furthermore, it is worth noting that wives' employment status exerts no effect on husbands' attitudes. As seen in Model 2 of Table 4.11, the regression coefficients of wives' employment status are not statistically significant. In other words, a husband's attitudes do not differ whether his wife is in or out of employment. We can therefore argue that a husband's attitudes to partnership and family are strongly affected by a couple's financial factors.

Table 4.11 Results of logistic latent class regression for husbands

	Model 1		Model 2		Model 3		Model 4	
	Neutral/ conservative	Progressive/ conservative	Neutral/ conservative	Progressive/ conservative	Neutral/ conservative	Progressive/ conservative	Neutral/ conservative	Progressive/ conservative
Covariate	Coefficient	Coefficient	Coefficient	Coefficient	Coefficient	Coefficient	Coefficient	Coefficient
Constant	0.35*	0.52*	0.64*	0.69*	0.26*	1.62*	1.03*	0.64*
Duration of marriage+								
Less than 3 years	4.48*	2.20*	3.93*	1.84*	2.53*	1.15*	1.64*	1.72*
4–6 years	2.34	0.83	2.15	1.18	1.24	0.16	1.13	0.64
7–9 years	2.41	1.11	1.28	1.21	1.30	0.53	1.04	0.48
10–12 years	0.54	0.36	0.42	1.01	0.93	0.17	0.81	0.10
13–15 years	0.19	0.16	0.06	0.04	−0.02	−0.07	−0.07	−0.09
(16 years–)								
Birth cohort								
Before 1959	−1.98	−1.97	−1.55	−0.21	0.59	1.38	0.18	0.83
(1960–1964)								
1965–1969	0.76	−0.63	−1.76	0.01	0.86	1.46	0.97	0.70
1970–1974	−2.27	−1.59	−0.68	−0.34	−0.75	−1.09	−0.09	−0.88
After 1975	−3.01	−1.64	−1.10	−1.12	−1.69	−1.58	−0.39	−1.82
The number of children ever-born+								
Childless	−0.01	−0.77	−0.65	0.84	0.15	−1.48		
1 child	0.38	0.50	0.07	−0.28	−0.37	−0.35		
(2 children or more)								

(continued)

Table 4.11 (continued)

	Model 1		Model 2		Model 3		Model 4	
	Neutral/ conservative	Progressive/ conservative	Neutral/ conservative	Progressive/ conservative	Neutral/ conservative	Progressive/ conservative	Neutral/ conservative	Progressive/ conservative
Covariate	Coefficient	Coefficient	Coefficient	Coefficient	Coefficient	Coefficient	Coefficient	Coefficient
Age at marriage								
(Under 23)								
24–26	−0.82	−0.02	−0.35	−0.90	−1.24	−0.80	−0.51	−0.73
27–29	−0.42	−0.20	−0.06	−0.78	−0.93	−0.55	−0.53	−0.17
30–32	0.32	−1.17	0.37	−0.87	−1.18	−0.97	−0.49	−0.60
33–35	−1.94	−0.02	−0.75	−1.91	−1.80	−0.24	−1.51	−0.50
Over 36	2.69	−3.50	−4.59	−1.99	−0.54	−1.64	−1.61	−0.91
Husband's income+								
(Less than 4,000,000 yen)								
4,000,000–7,990,000 yen	−1.49*	−0.44*	−0.14*	−0.90*	−1.54**	−1.17*	−0.78*	−0.64*
8,000,000 yen	0.42	0.25	0.29	0.20	0.53	0.25	0.04	0.11
Wife's income+								
No income	0.29	−0.25			0.19	−0.56	0.30	−0.57
(Less than 1,000,000 yen)								
1,000,000–2,990,000 yen	0.05	0.06			0.55	1.36	0.22	0.60
3,000,000 yen	2.17*	2.30*			1.69**	2.38**	0.76*	1.60*

(continued)

Table 4.11 (continued)

	Model 1		Model 2		Model 3		Model 4	
	Neutral/ conservative	Progressive/ conservative	Neutral/ conservative	Progressive/ conservative	Neutral/ conservative	Progressive/ conservative	Neutral/ conservative	Progressive/ conservative
Covariate	Coefficient	Coefficient	Coefficient	Coefficient	Coefficient	Coefficient	Coefficient	Coefficient
Wife's employment status+								
(Not working)								
Part-time worker			−0.35	−0.09				
Full-time worker			2.66	0.24				
Childbirth experience+								
(Not have a child)					−0.70	−1.15		
Had a child								
Childbearing experience by Birth order+								
Not have a child							0.03	0.38
Had a first child							−0.92	−1.08
(Had a second or higher-order child)								
Log-likelihood	−3924.68		−3929.81		−3924.5868		−3923.9536	
BIC	8251.17		8248.05		8304.565		8276.5108	
N	473		473		473		473	

Parentheses are reference categories
+ is a time-varying variable
Source the Japanese generations and gender survey
$^{*}p < 0.10$; $^{**}p < 0.05$; $^{***}p < 0.01$

Interestingly, the experience of having a child does not have a significant impact on husbands' attitudes. Neither the odds ratio of the neutral over the conservative group nor that of the progressive over the conservative group was affected by having a child (see Table 4.11, Model 3). Moreover, as far as the result of Model 4 in Table 4.11 shows, the birth order of a child also has no bearing on husbands' attitudes. In other words, an impact that having a child makes on husbands' attitudes does not differ between first-order birth and higher-order birth. Thus, we can argue that, for husbands, even the experience of bringing a life into the world does not bring ideational changes with it.

Now let us turn to the result of the wives' analysis in Table 4.12. As with the husbands' analysis, the demographic variables do not, as a whole, reveal a conspicuous effect on wives' attitudes. The coefficient of wives who got married over age 36 is statistically significant, indicating that long-delayed marriage increases the odds ratio of the neutral over the conservative group (see Table 4.12, Model 1). In addition, birth cohorts also exert an effect on wives' attitudes. Unlike the figures for their husbands in Table 4.11, the odds ratio of the neutral over the conservative group of wives in Table 4.12 is greater for younger birth cohorts, although this change may be due to an age effect or to a cohort effect; it is certain that value-orientation is not constant throughout one's life. Nevertheless, the remaining demographic variables do not yield significant coefficients in the model.

As for wives' annual income, a higher salary leads to a significant increase in the proportion of women belonging to the neutral and progressive groups. Compared with wives who earned less than 1,000,000 yen a year, those who obtained more than or equal to 3,000,000 yen yielded a 2.6 times greater odds ratio of the neutral over the conservative category. Similarly, the odds ratio of the progressive over the conservative category was 1.7 times higher for wives whose annual income exceeded 3,000,000 yen. In contrast, the level of husbands' income does not produce a significant coefficient. Furthermore, wives' employment status likewise shows no significant effect on their attitudes (see Table 4.12, Model 2). In short, value-commitment does not differ between wives in or out of employment. We can therefore argue that women's attitudes towards partnership and family relations are affected by their own earning levels.

The interesting point here is that the experience of childbearing, which had no impact on the value-orientation of husbands, played an important role in wives' value-orientation. More specifically, the odds ratio of the neutral over the conservative group reduced by 40 % after women gave birth to a child (see Table 4.12, Model 3). Likewise, this experience decreased the odds ratio of progressive over conservative wives by 60 %. Furthermore, the influence of childbearing varied between birth orders. Compared with women who bore a second child, those who gave birth to a first child had an 85 % lower odds ratio of the neutral over the conservative category (see Table 4.12, Model 4). Similarly, the odds ratio of progressive over conservative women fell by 84 % when they experienced a first childbirth. It, therefore, follows that becoming a parent makes women have more conservative ideas about partnership and family. Moreover, this effect is limited to mothers only.

Table 4.12 Results of logistic latent class regression for wives

	Model 1		Model 2		Model 3		Model 4	
	Neutra/ conservative	Progressive/ conservative	Neutra/ conservative coefficient	Progressive/ conservative	Neutra/ conservative	Progressive/ conservative	Neutral/ conservative	Progressive/ conservative
Covariate	Coefficient	Coefficient	Coefficient	Coefficient	Coefficient	Coefficient	Coefficient	Coefficient
Constant	−9.77*	0.32*	−1.15*	0.87*	−1.77*	0.22*	−1.91*	1.02*
Duration of marriage+								
Less than 3 years	0.44	0.19	0.17	4.22	2.32	2.16	0.04	0.19
4–6 years	1.30	0.13	0.72	1.90	1.45	1.87	0.21	1.37
7–9 years	0.44	0.65	0.66	0.86	0.38	0.97	1.36	0.58
10–12 years	1.18	0.42	0.28	0.38	0.31	0.44	1.73	1.28
13–15 years	−1.07	0.51	0.43	0.26	−0.21	0.32	1.82	1.28
(16 years–)								
Birth cohort								
Before 1959	−2.20	0.29	−0.82	−0.56	−0.41	−0.69	−0.72	−2.43
(1960–1964)								
1965–1969	0.31*	0.30	0.41*	0.45	0.47*	0.30	1.15*	1.93
1970–1974	0.42**	1.36	0.93*	1.51	1.29*	0.53	1.57*	1.48
After 1975	0.35**	0.45	0.88*	0.82	0.58*	0.78	1.25**	1.97
The number of children ever-born+								
Childless	0.87	0.88	0.16	0.74	0.89	0.12		
1 child	−0.08	−0.27	0.47	0.28	0.02	0.33		

(continued)

Table 4.12 (continued)

	Model 1		Model 2		Model 3		Model 4	
	Neutra/ conservative	Progressive/ conservative	Neutra/ conservative coefficient	Progressive/ conservative	Neutra/ conservative	Progressive/ conservative	Neutral/ conservative	Progressive/ conservative
Covariate	Coefficient	Coefficient	Coefficient	Coefficient	Coefficient	Coefficient	Coefficient	Coefficient
(2 children or more)								
Age at marriage								
(Under 23)								
24–26	−0.64	0.50	−0.66	0.45	−0.80	0.65	−0.80	0.33
27–29	0.13	0.28	−0.22	0.14	−0.41	0.29	−0.60	0.30
30–32	−2.59	0.67	−0.05	0.70	0.60	0.18	1.58	3.04
33–35	−0.51	1.03	−0.24	0.86	−0.81	0.43	1.72	3.43
Over 36	1.14**	1.52	1.44*	0.94	1.65*	0.17	1.30**	1.39
Husband's income+								
(Less than 4,000,000 yen)								
4,000,000–7,990,000 yen	−0.13	0.14	−0.34	−0.68	−0.32	0.04	−0.27	−0.45
8,000,000 yen	−3.54	−0.28	−0.52	−0.68	−0.70	−0.36	−3.71	−3.52
Wife's income+								
No Income	−2.28***	−0.59**			−0.34**	−0.22**	−2.70**	−2.20**
(Less than 1,000,000 yen)								
1,000,000-2,990,000 yen	0.13	0.16			0.14	0.17	0.03	−0.09
3,000,000 yen	0.98**	0.54*			1.65**	0.33**	2.41**	2.95**

(continued)

Table 4.12 (continued)

	Model 1		Model 2		Model 3		Model 4	
	Neutra/ conservative	Progressive/ conservative	Neutra/ conservative coefficient	Progressive/ conservative	Neutra/ conservative	Progressive/ conservative	Neutral/ conservative	Progressive/ conservative
Covariate	Coefficient	Coefficient	Coefficient	Coefficient	Coefficient	Coefficient	Coefficient	Coefficient
Wife's employment status+								
(Not working)								
Part-time worker			0.62	−0.55				
Full-time worker			0.22	0.65				
Childbirth experience+								
(Not have a child)								
Had a child					−0.99*	−0.89**		
Childbearing experience by birth order+								
Not have a child							0.05	0.51
Had a first child							−1.92**	−1.82**
(Had a second or higher-order child)								
Log-likelihood	−4923.16		−4923.28		−4922.91		−4928.24	
BIC	10,292.51		10278.80		10,305.96		10,302.67	
N	731		731		731		731	

Parentheses are reference categories
\+ is a time-varying variable
Source The Japanese generations and gender survey
$*p < 0.10$; $**p < 0.05$; $***p < 0.01$

4.10 Conclusion

The primary aim of this chapter was to investigate the influence of economic and ideational factors on fertility behaviour in Japan. First of all, we found that neither husbands' nor wives' incomes affected the probability of having a child. This suggests that the direct and indirect costs of rearing children play no significant role in determining fertility behaviour. This being the case, we may conclude that the economic theory of fertility cannot entirely explain Japanese fertility behaviour.

Second, we were able to identify that female employment status has a clear influence on fertility behaviour. Compared with wives who are out of employment, wives in employment showed a lower probability of having a child. Furthermore, this effect was still significant, even when the effect of a husband's participation in housework was controlled. These findings suggest that the conflict between family and employment plays a crucial role in low fertility in Japan. Moreover, our results indicate that this conflict has hardly been resolved only by the coordination of domestic chores between a husband and wife. We can therefore argue that more effective public policies for improving the work–life balance are necessary to prevent a further decline in Japanese fertility.

Third, our results showed that the levels of couples' incomes affect their attitudes towards partnership and family relations. More specifically, a higher-salaried wives were less conservative, whereas husbands with a medium level income had a more conservative attitudes. These findings indicated that an earning power has an influence on one's ideas on partnership and family relations.

Fourth, our analysis found that attitudinal factors have an impact on fertility behaviour. The risk of having a child is smaller for couples with progressive attitudes than those with conservative attitudes. The effect of ideational factors was particularity salient for husbands whose wives were not employed and for wives in full-time employment. Similarly, wives' attitudes had a great influence on fertility behaviour when they were in full-time employment. It is therefore safe to say that Japanese fertility behaviour is affected by ideational factors.

At the same time, however, we found that wives tend to become more conservative in their attitudes after giving birth; this tendency is particularly apparent after the birth of their first child. In short, values and attitudes exert an influence on determining married couples' reproductive behaviour in contemporary Japan. Yet, their values and attitude are, at the same time, affected by childbirth as well. In this regard, children are still important components of one's family, and having a child is a determining and influential life event for Japanese women. Ariès (1980) claims that King "Child" has been dethroned in the contemporary family. However, as far as our analysis shows, the regime of King "Child" does not seem to have been overthrown at all, and King "Couple" has not yet succeeded to the throne in Japan.

References

Ahn, N., & Mira, P. (2001). Job bust, baby bust?: Evidence from Spain. *Journal of Population Economics, 14*, 505–521.

Andorka, R. (1978). *The determinants of fertility in advanced societies*. London: Methuen.

Ariès, P. (1980). Two successive motivations for the declining birth rate in the west. *Population and Development Review, 6*, 645–650.

Axinn, W. G., & Thornton, A. (1992). The relationship between cohabitation and divorce: Selectivity or causal influence? *Demography, 29*, 357–374.

Balbo, N., Billari, F. C., & Mills, M. (2013). Fertility in advanced societies: A review of research. *European Journal of Population, 29*, 1–38.

Becker, G. S. (1960). An economic analysis of fertility. In *Demographic and economic change in developed countries*, edited by Universities-National Bureau Committee for Economic Research (pp. 209–231). Princeton: Princeton University Press.

Becker, G. S. (1975). *Human capital: A theoretical and empirical analysis, with special reference to education*. Chicago: University of Chicago Press.

Becker, G. S. (1976). *The economic approach to human behavior*. Chicago: The University of Chicago Press.

Becker, G. S. (1981). *A treatise on the family*. Cambridge, Massachusetts: Harvard University Press.

Becker, G. S., & Lewis, H. G. (1973). On the interaction between quantity and quality of children. *Journal of Political Economy, 81*, S279–S288.

Blake, J. (1967). Income and reproductive motivation. *Population Studies, 21*, 185–206.

Blake, J. (1968). Are babies consumer durables? A critique of the economic theory of reproductive motivation. *Population Studies, 22*, 5–25.

Bongaarts, J. (1976). Intermediate fertility variables and marital fertility rates. *Population Studies, 30*, 227–241.

Bongaarts, J. (1978). A framework of analyzing the proximate determinants of fertility. *Population and Development Review, 4*, 105–132.

Bongaarts, J., & Feeney, G. (1998). On the quantum and tempo of fertility. *Population and Development Review, 24*, 271–291.

Bongaarts, J., & Feeney, G. (2000). On the quantum and tempo of fertility: Reply. *Population and Development Review, 26*, 560–564.

Brodmann, S., Esping-Andersen, G., & Güell, M. (2007). When fertility is bargained: Second births in Denmark and Spain. *European Sociological Review, 23*, 599–613.

Bulatao, R. A., & Lee, R. D. (1983). A framework for the study of fertility determinants. In R. Bulatao & R. D. Lee (Eds.), *Determinants of fertility in developing countries* (pp. 1–26). New York: Academic Press.

Bumpass, L. (1969). Age at marriage as a variable in socio-economic differentials in fertility. *Demography, 6*, 45–54.

Bumpass, L., & Mburugu, E. K. (1977). Age at marriage and completed family size. *Social Biology, 24*, 31–37.

Busfield, J. (1972). Age at marriage and family size: Social causation and social selection hypotheses. *Journal of Biosocial Science, 4*, 117–134.

Butz, W., & Ward, M. (1979). The emergence of counter-cyclical US fertility. *American Economic Review, 69*, 318–328.

Cabinet Office. (2009). *National opinion survey on social life*. Tokyo: Cabinet Office.

Caldwell, J. C. (1982). *Theory of fertility decline*. New York: Academic Press.

Caldwell, J. C. (2006). *Demographic transition theory*. Dordrecht: Springer.

Davis, K., & Blake, J. (1956). Social structure and fertility: An analytic framework. *Economic Development and Cultural Change, 4*, 211–235.

Easterlin, R. A. (1971). Does human fertility adjust to the environment? *American Economic Review, 61*, 399–407.

Easterlin, R. A. (1978). The economics and sociology of fertility. In C. Tilly (Ed.), *Historical studies of changing fertility* (pp. 57–134). Princeton: Princeton University Press.
Elder, G. H. (1977). *Children of the great depression: Social change in life experience*. Chicago: University of Chicago Press.
Engelhardt, H., & Prskawetz, A. (2004). On the changing correlation between fertility and female employment over space and time. *European Journal of Population, 20*, 35–62.
Engelhardt, H., Kögel, T., & Prskawetz, A. (2004). Fertility and women's employment reconsidered: A macro-level time-series analysis for developed countries, 1960–2000. *Population Studies, 58*, 109–120.
Ermisch, J. (1970). Time costs, aspirations, and the effect of economic growth on german fertility. *Oxford Bulletin of Economics and Statistics, 42*, 125–144.
Ermisch, J. (1979). The relevance of the "easterlin hypothesis" and "new home economics" to fertility movement in great Britain. *Population Studies, 33*, 39–58.
Friedlander, S., & Silver, M. (1967). A quantitative study of the determinants of fertility behavior. *Demography, 4*, 30–70.
Fukuda, N. (2003a). Comparing family-friendly policies in Japan and Europe: Are we in the same or in a different league? *Journal of Population and Social Security, 1*, 31–45.
Fukuda, N. (2003b). Governmental support for families with children: Japan and Europe. *Journal of Population Problems, 59*, 7–26.
Gauthier, A. H. (1996). *The state and the family*. Oxford: Clarendon Press.
Guo, S., & Fraser, M. W. (2014). *Propensity score analysis: Statistical methods and applications*. Thousand Oaks, California: Sage Publications.
Hagenaars, J. A. (1993). *Loglinear models with latent variables*. Thousand Oaks, California: Sage Publications.
Hagenaars, J. A., & McCutcheon, A. L. (2002). *Applied latent class analysis*. Cambridge: Cambridge University Press.
Hashimoto, M. (1974). Economics of postwar fertility in Japan. *Journal of Political Economy, 82*, S170–S194.
Hashimoto, M. (1980). Demand for children in Japan during modernization. *Research in Population Economics, 2*, 295–320.
Hirschman, C., & Rindfuss, R. R. (1982). The sequence and timing of family formation events in Asia. *American Sociological Review, 47*, 660–680.
Hochschild, Arlie Russell, & Machung, Anne. (2003). *The second shift*. New York: Penguin Books.
Hodge, R. W., & Ogawa, N. (1991). *Fertility change in contemporary Japan*. Chicago: University of Chicago Press.
Hoem, B. (1993). The compatibility of employment and childbearing in contemporary Sweden. *Acta Sociologica, 36*, 101–120.
Hoem, B., & Hoem, J. (1989). The impact of women's employment on second and third birth in modern Sweden. *Population Studies, 43*, 47–67.
Jones, E. F. (1981). The impact of women's employment on marital fertility in the U.S., 1970–75. *Population Studies, 35*, 161–173.
Joshi, H. (1998). The opportunity cost of childbearing: More than mothers' business. *Journal of Population Economics, 11*, 161–183.
Kögel, T. (2004). Did the association between fertility and female employment within OECD countries really change its sign? *Journal of Population Economics, 17*, 45–65.
Kravdal, Ø. (1992). The weak impact of female labour force participation on Norwegian third-birth rates. *European Journal of Population, 8*, 247–263.
Kohler, H. P., Billari, F. C., & Ortega, J. A. (2002). The emergence of lowest-low fertility in Europe during the 1990s. *Population and Development Review, 28*, 641–680.
Murphy, M. (1993a). The contraceptive pill and women's employment as factors in fertility change in Britain 1963–1980: A challenge to the conventional view. *Population Studies, 47*, 221–247.

Murphy, M. (1993b). Time-series approaches to the analysis of fertility change. In M. Ní Bhrolcháin (Ed.), *New perspectives of fertility in Britain* (pp. 51–66). London: OPCS.

Mincer, J. (1963). Market prices, opportunity costs and income effects. In C. F. Christ, M. Friedman, L. A. Goodman, Z. Griliches, A. C. Harberger, N. Liviatan, J. Mincer, Y. Mundlak, M. Nerlove, D. Patinkin, L. G. Telser & H. Theil (Eds.), *Measurement in econometrics: Studies in mathematical economics and econometrics in memory of Yehuda Grunfeld* (pp. 67–82). Stanford: Stanford University Press.

Ministry of Education, Culture, Sports, Science and Technology. (Various years). *School basic survey*. Tokyo: Ministry of Education, Culture, Sports, Science and Technology.

Ministry of Health, Labour and Welfare. (2012). *Basic survey on wage structure*. Tokyo: Ministry of Health, Labour and Welfare.

Ministry of Health, Labour and Welfare. (Various years). *Vital statistics*. Tokyo: Ministry of Health, Labour and Welfare. Ministry of Internal Affairs and Communications. (2012). *Survey on time use and leisure activities*. Tokyo: Ministry of Internal Affairs and Communications.

Ministry of Internal Affairs and Communications. (2012). *Survey on time use and leisure activities*. Tokyo: Ministry of Internal Affairs and Communications.

National Institute of Population and Social Security Research. (Various years). *Japanese fertility survey*. Tokyo: Health and Welfare Statistics Association.

Osawa, M. (1988). Working mothers: Changing patterns of employment and fertility in Japan. *Economic Development and Cultural Change, 36*, 623–650.

Raftery, A. E. (1995). Bayesian model selection in social research. In P. V. Marsden (Ed.), *Sociological methodology* (pp. 111–163). Oxford: Basil Blackwell.

Retherford, R., & Ogawa, N. (2006). Japan's baby bust: Cause, implications, and policy responses. In F. R. Harris (Ed.), *The baby bust: Who will do the work? who will pay the taxes?* (pp. 5–47). Lanham: Rowman & Littlefielf Publishers.

Retherford, R., Ogawa, N., & Sakamoto, S. (1996). Values and fertility change in Japan. *Population Studies, 50*, 5–25.

Ryder, N. B. (1965). The cohort as a concept in the study of social change. *American Sociological Review, 30*, 843–861.

Vermunt, J. K. (1997). *Log-linear models for event histories*. London: Sage Publications.

Waite, L. J., Goldscheider, F. K., & Witsberger, C. (1986). Non-family living and the erosion of traditional family orientations among young adults. *American Sociological Review, 51*, 541–554.

Weller, R. H. (1977). Wife's employment and cumulative family size in the United States, 1960 and 1970. *Demography, 14*, 43–65.

Westoff, C. F., & Ryder, N. B. (1977). *Contraceptive revolution*. Princeton: Princeton University Press.

Westoff, C. F., Hammerslough, C. R., & Paul, C. (1987). The potential impact of improvements in contraception and fertility in western countries. *European Journal of Population, 3*, 7–32.

Wilkinson, M. (1973). An econometric analysis of fertility in Sweden, 1870–1965. *Econometrica, 41*, 633–642.

Willis, R. J. (1973). A new approach to the economic theory of fertility behavior. *Journal of Political Economy, 81*, S14–S64.

Willis, R. J. (1987). The family. What have we learned from the economics of the family? *American Economic Review, 77*, 68–81.

Yamamura, K., & Hanley, S. (1975). Ichi hime, Ni Tarô: Education aspirations and the decline of fertility in Postwar Japan. *Journal of Japanese Studies, 2*, 83–125.

Zuanna, G. D. (2004). The Banquet of Aeolus: A familistic interpretattion of Italy's lowest low fertility. In G. Dalla Zuanna & G. A. Micheli (Eds.), *Strong family and low fertility: A paradox?: New perspectives in interpreting contemporary family and reproductive behaviour* (pp. 105–125). Dordrecht: Kluwer Academic Publishers.

Chapter 5
Stability and Change in Value-Orientations

5.1 Introduction

In this chapter, we will investigate attitudinal changes between generations in Japan. As put forward in the previous chapters, ideational factors have affected Japanese marriage and fertility behaviour. More specifically, people who held progressive and individualistic attitudes showed a lower risk of getting married and giving birth to children. It would, however, be premature to conclude that ideational factors played a key role in determining patterns of marriage and childbearing in Japan over the past few decades. Admittedly, we found in the previous chapters that a transition from one stage to another stage in an individual life course was affected by value-orientation. To be concrete, we saw that marriage and childbearing behaviour were affected by individual values and attitudes. However, we must bear in mind that this holds true only for the Japanese population at the time of our survey. In other words, what we clarified is the mechanism of nuptial and childbearing behaviour at a specific point in historical time. As discussed in Chap. 2, a value shift is regarded as a long-lasting and continuous process (Ariès 1980; Lesthaeghe 1983). Thus, if Japanese marriage and fertility patterns have a bearing on ideational transformations, a persistent attitudinal change should be observed across generations. In other words, if different cohorts have different attitudes towards partnership and family, it may be more persuasively argued that ideational factors have an impact on marriage and fertility behaviour in Japan.

Taking this point into consideration, in this chapter we will examine whether ideational change can be identified between birth cohorts and temporal periods in Japan. In this chapter, we will first provide the theoretical review on the relation between socio-economic development and value-orientation. After explaining the data and methods used in this chapter, we will look at a difference in attitudes from a viewpoint of cohorts and periods. Finally, we will examine attitudinal change between generations in Japan by employing Hierarchical Age-Period-Cohort (HAPC) analysis.

N. Fukuda, *Marriage and Fertility Behaviour in Japan*,
DOI 10.1007/978-981-10-0294-6_5

5.2 Socio-economic Development and Value Change

Although various descriptions have been given regarding values and attitudes in contemporary industrialized societies, their features can be summarized in two points (Bauman 2000; Beck et al. 1994; Bell 1976; Inglehart 1990; Inglehart and Baker 2000). The first point holds that the regulating influence of traditional norms and customs upon individual actions has been weakening gradually over time. As a result, ideological pluralism has spread and diverse lifestyles have gained greater tolerance in societies. At the same time, this transformation allows people to enjoy a high degree of freedom of choice where personal behaviour is concerned. The second of these points identifies a concurrent manifestation of individuals' strong preoccupation with and aspiration towards the pursuit of self-expression and self-fulfilment in society. This trend allows people to have more self-reliant and individualistic preferences and enables them to place significant weight on their own goal attainment in the social sphere.

Although the dissemination of these values and attitudes varies from one society to another, it is commonly acknowledged that this ideational shift has a tight connection to socio-economic development (Inglehart 1977; Inglehart and Welzel 2005; Halman et al. 2008). As discussed in Chap. 2, since a less developed society holds fewer socio-economic resources, its members' existence can be critically threatened by behaviour that deviates from conventional norms and customs. In these societies, therefore, an individual's actions need to conform to conventional rules, and through the placement of these tight controls on individuals' actions, the community is able to allocate its scarce resources in an optimal way and to secure its continuing existence (Wrigley 1978). With the attainment of economic growth and increased social security, however, the constraints of conventional norms placed on human actions are relaxed. A high productive capacity caused by economic growth can produce a vast amount of socio-economic resources, which leads to a society's emancipation from the existential threats of material scarcity. In addition, the implementation of public welfare programmes serves to reduce the economic insecurity previously felt by many people. As a result, human actions no longer need to be tightly regulated by conventional customs and norms, and people can enjoy freedom of choice in their behaviour.

In addition, socio-economic development can transform the structure of human needs. The centre of human desires shifts from material needs to personal self-fulfilment, in parallel with the enhancement of physical prosperity (Inglehart 1977, 1990). More specifically, in earlier stages of economic development, the satisfaction of material needs (lower-order needs) has the highest priority in the order of human desire; at these stages, sustenance for daily existence is relatively scarce. However, as a society develops materially and economically, the individual's priority of needs shifts to personal self-fulfilment and self-expression (higher-order needs); at this stage, people do not have to worry about the scarcity of sustenance. Following this developmental schema of human needs, we can see that the recent economic prosperity of industrialized countries has reached the stage where self-expression and self-fulfilment dominate (Maslow 1970).

Looking at socio-economic development in Japan, we can identify the sufficient material conditions that foster a consciousness that accepts diverse lifestyles and seeks self-fulfilment. While Japan lagged behind other developed countries somewhat in living standards a couple of decades ago, it now matches them. For instance, as seen in Graph 5.1, the Japanese GDP (per capita converted by the purchasing power parity) tripled from 12,948 US dollars in 1970 to 30,760 US dollars in 2011 (OECD iLibrary). Hence, Japanese society enjoys unprecedented material affluence.

Moreover, due to the development of social security programmes, considerable amounts of public benefits are distributed in kind and cash in Japan. As seen in Graph 5.2, although the percentage of public spending in Japan's GDP stood at only 10.2 % in 1980, this figure had doubled to 22.2 % by 2010. This percentage

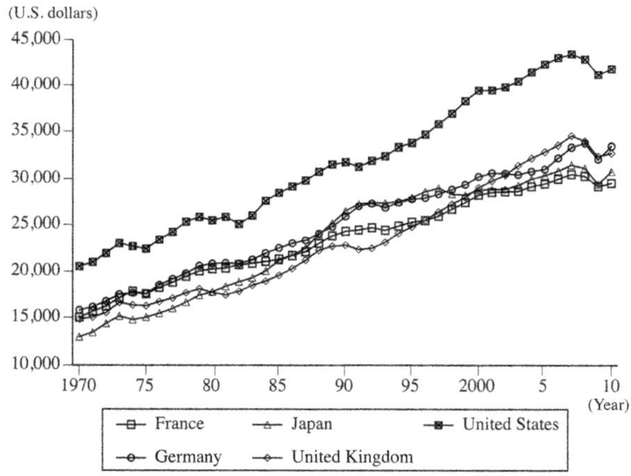

Graph 5.1 GDP per capita, selected countries. *Note* US dollars are converted by the purchasing power parity. *Source* OECD iLibrary

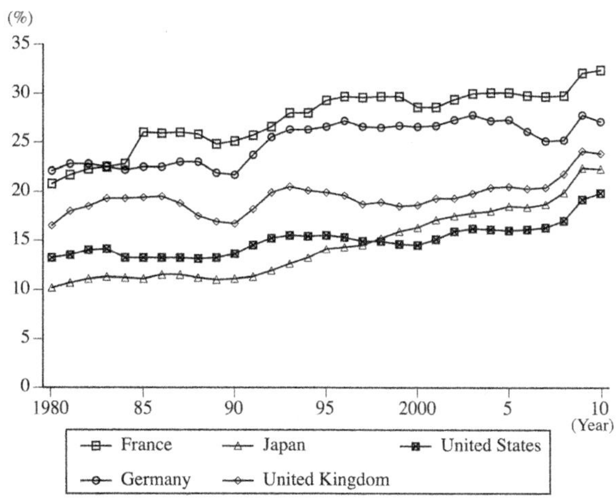

Graph 5.2 Percentage of public-spending per GDP, selected countries. *Source* OECD iLibrary

Graph 5.3 The percentage of respondents who agreed that marriage was an outdated institution. *Source* Inglehart and Basañez (2010)

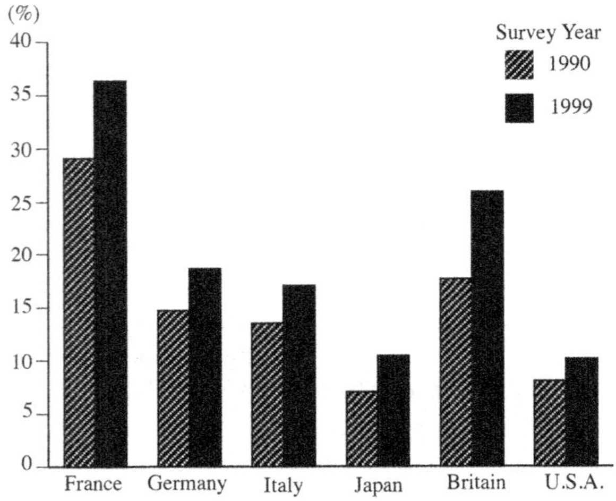

is well in line with public-spending figures in European countries. Admittedly, a rise in the number of people in need increases the amount of welfare spending. Thus, an increase in public spending may not necessarily lead to reducing anxieties surrounding social issues and enhancing people's sense of security. At the same time, it cannot be, however, denied that Japan has reached the stage where its population seeks freedom of choice, with individuals displaying a strengthening desire for self-fulfilment and self-expression from an economic and material viewpoint. Hence, it seems possible that less conventional and more individualistic attitudes towards partnership and family relationship are gradually gaining in popularity in Japan.

It is, however, debatable whether socio-economic development immediately leads to transformations in human value-orientation and behaviour in society (Haller 2002). In fact, the World Value Surveys illustrate that developed countries do not always experience the same ideational change. For instance, the percentage of respondents who agreed that marriage was an outdated institution reached 36.3% in France in 1999, while that stood at only 10.4 % in Japan (see Graph 5.3). Moreover, although France and Britain exhibit a salient increase in the percentage from 1990 until 1999, such a change is not seen in the remaining countries. This evidence clearly shows that an ideational change differs between developed countries.

The reason for this diverse value shift is, first of all, that one's values and attitudes tend to be moulded to a considerable degree before reaching adulthood and are not likely to change substantially thereafter (Newson and Richerson 2009). Generally speaking, a society constantly accepts newly-born members as long as it continues to exist; its older generations work to inculcate their traditional values in succeeding generations, thus giving a succession of young strangers a sense of membership in their society. Without this type of orientation, a society would cease to exist for lack of integration. In sociological terms, this process is called "socialization", which is an indispensable component for making a society viable by coordinating human behaviours (Durkheim 1956; Merton 1968). Admittedly, socialization is performed by several agents such as peer groups, family members and schools, but the interaction between children and parents has a primary and powerful influence on the value formation of infant children (Parsons and Bales 1955). In short, older generations transmit values and beliefs which they deem to be desirable upon younger generations through primary socialization within the family. Accordingly, values formed in the minds of children in a formative period have fundamentally traditional and conventional characteristics. Hence, as long as conventional values and beliefs are reproduced in younger generations through primary socialization, it follows that ideational changes between generations are quite unlikely. We should not, however, forget that a family is not the only agent of socialization that one encounters in life. For instance, human beings are also socialized through many interactions between peer groups at school and colleagues in the workplace. Such first-hand experiences in adolescence and young adulthood may modify or change one's values and norms, which were formerly moulded in childhood in one's family. Hence, this secondary socialization can exert enough influence to cause individuals to adopt new values or beliefs based on first-hand experiences in adolescence and young adulthood. When this happens, younger generations may acquire values and norms differing from those transmitted through primary socialization within the natal family. In particular, if values and beliefs acquired in adolescence and young adulthood tend to find harmonious acceptance within affluent and secure societies, people's behaviour is more likely to be oriented towards the acceptance of diverse lifestyles and the realization of self-fulfilment. In this case, socio-economic development causes ideational change in the way that Inglehart (1990, 1995, 1997, 2003) described. Yet, we must keep in mind that it is difficult to discern which of the primary or secondary socialization exerts more influence on one's value formation a priori. Hence, socio-economic development does not necessarily lead to ideational or attitudinal changes between generations.

Second, even if changes in human values and attitudes are observed in a cross-sectional survey, it is methodologically difficult to judge whether they are attributable to an attitudinal difference between generations. Generally speaking, variations on one's attitudes are composed of three factors: age effects, period effects and cohort effects (Glenn 2003; Yang 2008; Yang and Land 2006, 2008; Hobcraft and Preston 1985). The first of these factors, age effects, originates in the biological and social processes of human ageing. People undergo physiological transformations and accumulate social experiences as they grow up and shape their life course. As a result of this, individual values and attitudes may change and differ between ages. Period effects, the second of these three factors, are related to social environments and events such as economic depression and war. People who share the experience of such an episode at a point in historical time may change their values and beliefs temporarily. For instance, people living in a period of deep economic recession may hold a pessimistic attitude towards the future. Hence, period effects influence all age groups simultaneously within a specific time frame. Finally, cohort effects are ideational variations seen in a group of people who have experienced a life event such as birth or marriage in the same calendar years. People in the same birth cohort experience social changes or events at similar ages, exposing them to identical social conditions at the same stage of their life development. Consequently, individual values and attitudes are considerably homogeneous among the same birth cohort and heterogeneous among different birth cohorts. Although the word "cohort" is more often used than "generation" in the field of life-course studies, the two words are virtually interchangeable in terms of the meaning assigned to them.

On the theoretical side, it is necessary to discern the influence of these three factors on an attitudinal change, because age, period and cohort effects have different background causes and interpretations. In particular, since the analysis of people's attitudes is one of the most important purposes in a social survey, it is preferable to examine the strengths of these three effects separately. On the practical side, however, it is quite difficult to identify the extent to which each effect determines people's values and attitudes with a cross-sectional survey data (Mason et al. 1973). Indeed, empirical analyses have not always yielded consistent results with regard to age, period and cohort effects. To take, as an example, the World Value Surveys, Inglehart and Baker (2000) maintain that cohort effects play a crucial role in the value change of advanced Western countries. Yet, no unanimous consensus exists over this interpretation. Indeed, some scholars insist that age effects have a strong impact on attitudes in the developed countries (Tranter and Western 2003; Jagodzinski 1983), while others claim that period effects have a crucial bearing on the value change of these countries (Clarke et al. 1999).

The main reason for these inconsistent results is that age, period and cohort effects are not mutually independent. For the sake of simplification, let us assume that a change in attitudes is linearly associated with the three effects (Fienberg and Mason 1985). In this case, the model equation of attitudes is expressed in the following way:

$$\theta_{\mathrm{APC}} = \beta_0 + \beta_1\mathrm{A} + \beta_2\mathrm{P} + \beta_3\mathrm{C} \qquad (5.1)$$

where is θ_{APC} the attitude of a person i. Independent variables A, P and C designate age, period and cohort effects, respectively. Furthermore, β_1, β_2 and β_3 are coefficients of the independent variables; β_0 is a constant term. Seeing the coefficients in the equation at first glance, an investigation of the strengths of these three effects would appear to be simple and straightforward. In practice, however, an estimation of strengths becomes problematic, for the three variables are not linearly independent. More specifically, due to the fact that the three variables bear the relation "Cohort = Period-Age", any one of the three effects in Eq. (5.1) is equal to the sum or the difference of the other two effects. Hence, the functional form of Eq. (5.1) has the linear dependency, which makes it impossible to estimate the coefficients of the three variables separately with a cross-sectional survey. In short, the linear specification of age, period and cohort effects suffers from the so-called under-identification problem.

A number of techniques have been put forward in order to estimate age, period and cohort effects from cross-sectional data; their common feature is the placement of certain constraints on model Eq. (5.1) proposed by Fienberg and Mason (1985). Since the model equation has more parameters than it can calculate, auxiliary equations are introduced to estimate coefficients of independent variables properly. For instance, Sasaki and Suzuki (1987) estimate age, period and cohort effects on Japanese religious attitudes from a single cross-sectional survey, assuming that successive parameters change gradually. More specifically, they calculate coefficients of the three variables by imposing model Eq. (5.1) on the condition of minimizing the difference of adjacent parameters. In other words, by putting the equation under constraint conditions, these methods turn the state of under-identification in the linear specification into that of just-identification.

It is still, however, debatable whether these methods can properly estimate the parameters of age, period and cohort effects in the linear specification, for introduced auxiliary constraints do not always provide a guarantee for estimating proper parameters. In other words, the use of arbitrary and mechanical constraints may lead to biased estimators (Glenn 1989). Hence, drawing a distinction between age, period and cohort effects is theoretically important in the analysis of attitudinal change, but it is difficult, in practice, to estimate these three effects from a cross-sectional survey. This means, at the same time, that, even if attitudinal changes are observed from a survey in a single point of time, it is quite difficult to determine which of the three effects caused an ideational transformation. In short, even if attitudinal transformations are observed in a society at an economically prosperous stage, not all changes are attributable to cohort effects.

Third, a value shift may be caused by a change in social policy setting. As mentioned before, the level of security in a society is tightly linked to ideational change. This sense of security is, to a considerable extent, affected by governmental public support. For instance, generous welfare programmes such as health insurance and unemployment benefits give a strong feeling of stability and security to people's everyday lives. Thus, if social and welfare programmes change in their type, provision and eligibility, people are likely to sense a change in their level of security. This transformation in the sense of security consequently may lead to a change in values and attitudes. Hence, a value shift is affected not only by socio-economic development, but also by social policy setting.

On the other hand, where governmental public support is concerned, it has been posited that the patterns of welfare policy differ across advanced countries. For instance, Esping-Anderson (1990, 1999) classified contemporary welfare states into three types by using the degree of de-commodification and the principle of stratification as indicators of welfare system. More specifically, the former scale measures the extent to which a welfare state supports individuals and families independently of market participation, while the latter scale indicates the method by which a nation maintains the harmonization of its social classes. According to these two indicators, Esping-Anderson (1990, 1999) classifies the welfare systems of developed countries into liberal, social democratic and conservative (corporatist) regimes. According to his typology, a "liberal" welfare system is seen in states such as the USA and Australia, where there is less government intervention in health care and social security, both of which tend to be left to the market mechanism. In contrast, "social democratic" welfare states such as Sweden and Denmark make a strong governmental commitment to the well-being of people and the harmonization of social classes. Between these two types lies the corporatist welfare regime, where the level and coverage of governmental support is segmented by individual social status. Examples of this type of welfare state are Germany and Austria, where social insurance, pensions and benefits vary depending on occupational classes.

Beside Esping-Anderson's typology, many classifications have been hitherto proposed regarding governmental welfare policy in advanced countries (Fukuda 2003; Ferarra 1996; Gauthier 1996; Gauthier and Hatzius 1997; Gauthier and Philipov 2008; Gornick et al. 1997; Lewis 1992; Sainsbury 1994; Siaroff 1994; Thévenon 2011). To take an example, Goodman and Peng (1996) regard Japanese welfare policy as a hybrid of liberal and corporatist welfare regimes owing to the influence of traditional Confucianism and the post-war reforms of the USA It is of paramount importance to bear in mind here, however, that whatever the typology of state and policy is proposed, governmental support for an individual or for family life differs from nation to nation in its coverage, amount and eligibility. In other words, the level and quality of social security varies from one country to another. As mentioned earlier, the level of security in society has a strong bearing on ideational change. Moreover, the sense of security people feel is strongly related to the social policy their government implements. Taking these points into consideration, it seems possible that a different welfare regime brings a different sense of security, consequently leading to a different pattern of value change. In fact, Assave et al. (2013) find that policy and institution factors have a significant relation to attitudes towards family formation in European countries. Furthermore, Salles (2006) finds that a change of governmental policy in the former GDR (German Democratic Republic) was responsible for a change in marriage and fertility behaviour. Thus, due to differences in the coverage and amount of, and eligibility for, governmental welfare support, Japan may experience a different value shift from those experienced in Western developed countries. All told, it is necessary to examine empirically whether Japanese attitudes have changed between generations.

5.3 Data, Method, and Variables for the Analysis of Attitudinal Change

The present analysis used data gathered in the National Survey on Family in Japan (NSFJ), a nationwide repeated cross-sectional survey whose target population was married women in Japan. All respondents were selected by stratified probability sampling throughout Japan. The NSFJ was conducted in 1993 for the first time and is carried out once every five years. In the present analysis, we use data sets from the first to the fourth rounds of the NSFJ.[1] The response rates for this quinquennial survey were 80.6 % in its first year in 1993; 87.7 % in 1998; 76.9 % in 2003; and 76.7 % in 2008. We, in this analysis, selected married women between ages 20 and 79 at the time of each survey. The total number of respondents used in the analysis amounts to 16,016 women.

Admittedly, one's value-orientation may differ depending on one's marital status or gender. It may be, thus, difficult to plot the overall picture of Japanese attitudes from the quantitative analysis of married women. At the same time, however, it is extremely important to examine cohort, age and period effects on individual attitudes from a long perspective. As mentioned before, identification of the three effects is quite difficult to discern from the data of a single cross-sectional survey. In order to surmount this problem, we employed Hierarchical Age-Period-Cohort (HAPC) analysis in this study (Yang and Land 2006, 2008, 2013). As we will discuss in detail later, the HAPC method provides a great advantage by allowing us to estimate the three effects in a more flexible and less constrained way, although it requires a large pooled data from repeated cross-sectional surveys. Taking this feature of the method into consideration, it is most desirable to use data sets from as many rounds as possible of a repeated cross-sectional survey with identical items or questions posed in every round in order to measure respondents' values and attitudes. Unfortunately, data sets of such a type are quite rate, and the NSFJ is one of the very few surveys satisfying the aforementioned conditions. For these reasons, we decided to use the NSFJ data, although this meant that men could not be included our analysis. It should therefore be borne in mind that our results may be valid for women but not necessarily for men. In other words, we need to refrain from any over-generalization of our findings.

As mentioned previously, in the present study we employ Hierarchical Age-Period-Cohort (HAPC) analysis (Yang and Land 2006, 2008, 2013). The model of the HAPC analysis is expressed as follows:

$$Y_{ijk} = \beta_{0jk} + \beta_1 \mathrm{AGE}_{ijk} + \beta_2 \mathrm{AGE}^2_{ijk} + \beta_n X_{ijk} + e_{ijk} \tag{5.2}$$

where Y_{ijk} is a dependent variable at an individual i within cohort j and period k; $\beta_{0\,jk}$ is an intercept; AGE_{ijk} is the age of an individual i within cohort j and period k; β_1 is a parameter of the age; $\mathrm{AGE}^2{}_{ijk}$ is the age squared of an individual i within cohort j and period k; and β_2 is a parameter of the age squared. Furthermore, X_{ijk} is an independent variable other than the age of an individual i, and β_n is its parameter. Finally, e_{ijk} indicates an error term having the normal distribution with its mean 0 and variance σ^2. Since Eq. (5.2) is specified regarding the variables of each respondent, it is called the level-1 specification. In addition, the HAPC analysis specifies the following equation on the intercept:

$$\beta_{0\,jk} = \gamma_0 + \mu_{0j} + \upsilon_{0k} \tag{5.3}$$

[1]The data were provided under the Japanese Statistics Act. The author expresses great thanks to the National Institute of Population and Social Security Research for giving permission to use the data of the National Survey on Family in Japan.

Here, γ_0 is a constant term; μ_{0j} indicates the cohort effect or residual random effect of cohort j; υ_{0k} designates the period effect or residual random effect of period k. In addition, μ_{0j} and υ_{0k} are assumed to have the normal distribution with mean 0 and variance τ_{μ} and with mean 0 and variance τ_{υ}. This model specification is related not to individuals but to groups, that is to say, to cohorts and periods to which the respondents belong. Thus, Eq. (5.3) is called the level-2 specification. We treated the coefficients of the level-2 equation as the random effects model. The substitution of Eq. (5.3) into Eq. (5.2) then yields the combined model:

$$Y_{ijk} = \gamma_0 + \beta_1 \mathrm{AGE}_{ijk} + \beta_2 \mathrm{AGE}_{ijk}^2 + \beta_n X_{ijk} + \mu_{0j} + \upsilon_{0k} + e_{ijk} \quad (5.4)$$

As argued previously, it is quite difficult to examine age, cohort and period effects by applying an ordinary linear model to the data of a cross-sectional survey. In order to ressolve the problem, the HAPC method employs the pooled data of cross-sectional surveys and examines the effects of age, cohort and period with an application of multilevel analysis (Raudenbush and Bryk 2002).

Furthermore, we employ the inter-class correlation to evaluate the effects of cohorts and periods on respondents' attitudes. In concrete terms, the inter-class correlation ρ_1 is calculated in the following way:

$$\rho_1 = \frac{\sigma_2^2}{\sigma_1^2 + \sigma_2^2 + \sigma_3^2} \quad (5.5)$$

where σ_1^2 is the individual-level variance; σ_2^2 is the period-level variance; and σ_3^2 is the cohort-level variance. In Eq. (5.5), ρ_1 measures the extent of period effects on attitudes. By the same token, the inter-class correlation ρ_2 is expressed as follows:

$$\rho_2 = \frac{\sigma_3^2}{\sigma_1^2 + \sigma_2^2 + \sigma_3^2} \quad (5.6)$$

where σ_1^2 is the individual-level variance; σ_2^2 is the period-level variance; and σ_3^2 is the cohort-level variance. In Eq. (5.6), ρ_2 stands for the degree of birth cohort effects on attitudes.

5.3.1 Attitudinal Dependent Variables

The primary purpose of this study is to investigate an ideational change with data from the first to fourth round of the NSFJ. The dependent variable is, therefore, a respondent's attitude towards partnership and family relations. Since the NSFJ included many questions concerning respondents' views on marriage, children and family, we constructed a composite variable concerning their attitudes. The following nine opinion statements were presented for response in all four rounds of the NSFJ:

(1) A husband should work outside and a wife should devote herself to doing housework after marriage (**Husband–wife segregation**).
(2) Children should come first even if parents must make sacrifices in their own lives (**Children first**).
(3) It is better for a mother to devote herself to childrearing until her child reaches age three (**Mother child-rearing**).
(4) It is natural that boys are brought up to be manly and girls are brought up to be womanly (**Boys manly**).
(5) Marriage is socially accepted after a couple have children (**Marriage and children**).
(6) It is all right for a husband and wife to have different surnames (**Different surname**).
(7) A husband should prioritize his company's concerns above his family's concerns (**Company first**).
(8) Children should live with their aged parents under the same roof (**Co-residence with parents**).
(9) It is the duty of grown children to look after aged parents (**Care for parents**).

Each statement had four responding categories: (1) strongly agree; (2) agree; (3) disagree; and (4) strongly disagree. For each opinion statement, respondents were asked to choose the single responding category closest to their view at the time of the survey. Based on the responses to these statements, we created a scoring system that measures a respondent's attitudes towards partnership and family relationships. We gave a score of 1 to respondents for each statement where "strongly agree" was chosen; if respondents chose "agree", they were given a score of 2; when a respondent chose "disagree", she was given a score of 3; when a respondent chose "strongly disagree", her response received a score of 4. In short, we constructed a four-point evaluative scale. In this scale, a stronger disagreement with each opinion item yields a greater score.

Although the NSFJ has many opinion statements, they do not necessarily measure a single dimension of respondents' attitudes. It may be that attitudes to partnership and parent–child relations belong to a different dimension of value-orientation. In order to investigate the dimensional configuration of the aforementioned nine opinion items in the NSFJ, we conducted factor analysis on the nine items. As shown in Table 5.1, the opinion statements were classified into two dimensions.

To begin with, opinion items (1) "Husband–wife segregation", (3) "Mother child-rearing" and (4) "Boys manly" are strongly associated to factor 1. These three opinion statements are related to gender relations between husbands and wives, and sons and daughters. Hence, as the scores for these items become higher, respondents hold a less conventional and more progressive attitude towards gender relations. By contrast, lower scores indicate attitudes that are more traditional and conservative. In short, this scale measures the extent to which a respondent accepts conventional values in terms of gender relations. As for Cronbach's coefficient alpha, the three opinion items reached 0.695, having a

Table 5.1 Results of factor analysis for the NFSJ questions

Opinion statements	Factor loading	
	Factor 1	Factor 2
(1) Husband–wife segregation	0.589	0.262
(2) Children first	0.255	0.153
(3) Mother child-rearing	0.724	0.083
(4) Boys manly	0.548	0.320
(5) Marriage and children	0.314	0.433
(6) Different surname	−0.253	−0.261
(7) Company first	0.184	0.224
(8) Co-residence with parents	0.168	0.497
(9) Care for parents	0.078	0.460
Eigen value	2.767	1.052

$N = 16{,}016$

Opinion statements are as follows:

(1) A husband should work outside and a wife should devote herself to doing housework after marriage
(2) Children should come first even if parents must make sacrifices in their own lives
(3) It is better for a mother to devote herself to childrearing until her child reaches age three
(4) It is natural that boys are brought up to be manly and girls are brought up to be womanly
(5) Marriage is socially accepted after a couple have children
(6) It is all right for a husband and wife to have different surnames
(7) A husband should prioritize his company's concerns above his family's concerns
(8) Children should live with their aged parents under the same roof
(9) It is the duty of grown children to look after aged parents

Source The National Survey on Family in Japan.

sufficient reliability. Taking these results into consideration, we used the sum of the scores for items (1) "Husband–wife segregation", (3) "Mother child-rearing" and (4) "Boys manly" as a respondent's first attitudinal variable, labelling it as the respondent's "gender relation attitude". On the other hand, items (5) "Marriage and children", (8) "Co-residence with parents" and (9) "Care for parents" show a strong connection to factor 2. These opinion items are related to attitudes towards parent–child or couple–child relationships. In these items, a respondent's score increases with the level of importance she places on her own life over her parents and children. In other words, those women with higher scores have a more individualistic and self-centred attitude. Hence, these scores measure the extent to which a respondent cherishes individualistic values. Furthermore, Cronbach's coefficient alpha of the items stood at 0.583, showing a mildly consistent relation. Thus, the total value of the scores from items (5) "Marriage and children", (8) "Co-residence with parents" and (9) "Care for parents" was employed as a respondent's second attitudinal variable, which was termed "inter-generational relation attitudes". In the following part of this analysis, we will use these two composite variables as an indicator of a respondent's attitude.

5.3.2 Age, Cohort, and Period Variables

We shall examine the effects of age, cohort and period on attitudes. First of all, in order to examine the relation between age and attitudes, our analytical model includes a respondent's age as an independent variable. Furthermore, since the relation between the two factors may be nonlinear, the square term of a respondent's age is also included in our model. In this analysis, age and age squared are treated as a continuous variable.

Respondents' birth cohorts were divided into 13 groups: (1) Before 1924; (2) 1925–1929; (3) 1930–1934; (4) 1935–1939; (5) 1940–1944; (6) 1945–1949; (7) 1950–1954; (8) 1955–1959; (9) 1960–1964; (10) 1965–1969; (11) 1970–1974; (12) 1975–1979; and (13) 1980–. These cohorts include generations born from the pre-war period to those born in the so-called post-bubble economy after the 1990s. Since people in the same birth cohort experience a social change at similar ages or at the same stage of their life development, they seem to have a homogeneous value-orientation. In particular, it may be borne in mind that three major landmark periods occurred in post-war Japan: a miracle recovery from the Second World War; a period of unprecedented economic growth; and a heavy economic slump after the bubble economy in the 1980s. Different birth cohorts should have experienced these social changes at different life stages. It is, hence, expected that the impacts of these social transformations differ between birth cohorts, leading to the formation of different values and attitudes. In order to investigate the influence of this factor on human attitudes, our analytical model includes respondents' birth cohorts as an independent variable.

We employed four period categories: (1) the year 1993; (2) the year 1998; (3) the year 2003; and (4) the year 2008. These are the calendar years in which a round of the NFSJ was carried out. As put forward previously, since period effects are related to social environments at a point in historical time, these factors simultaneously affect all age groups living in such a social situation. In particular, Japan experienced turbulent economic conditions and a drastic transformation of its industrial structure in the "post-bubble" period after the late 1990s. It seems therefore likely that these harsh socio-economic circumstances engraved special features on people's attitudes.

As mentioned before, the HAPC analysis has independent variables in the level-1 and level-2 equations. Following the model specification of Yang and Land (2013), in our analysis, age and age squared were put in the level-1 equation, while birth cohort and period were employed as independent variables of the level-2 equation.

5.3.3 Other Variables

Two socio-economic and one demographic variable were included in our model. It is well known that individual values and attitudes differ between socio-economic positions. For instance, better-educated people may hold more progressive attitudes towards gender relations, whereas less-educated people may have a strong preference for traditional gender relations. In order to control the influence of such socio-economic factors on attitudes, we first employed a respondent's educational level as an explanatory variable of the level-1 equation. In concrete terms, the level of education which a respondent finally accomplished is classified into four categories: (1) primary or junior high school; (2) high school; (3) two-year junior college or vocational school; and (4) four-year university or higher. Second, our model included a spouse's (a husband's) annual income as an explanatory variable. This variable was divided into income groups: (1) less than 3,000,000 yen; (2) 3,000,000–6,000,000 yen; and (3) over 6,000,000 yen. These variables were used to control the effects of socio-economic factors on individual attitudes. At the same time, however, they also serve to control the composite effect on attitudinal transformation seen in birth cohorts and periods (Hauser 1970). For example, let us assume that a higher educational credential is connected to a less traditional attitude. In this case, a cohort comprised of many well-educated people will show more progressive characteristics, *ceteris paribus*, than that made up of few well-educated people. This is not because the two cohorts themselves have different attitudes (cohort effects), but because a pseudo-effect is caused by a difference in the proportion of well-educated people in the two groups. In other words, the characteristics of a group, *ceteris paribus*, change when the ratio of its components differs greatly. Hence, in order to examine the net effects that cohorts and periods themselves have on attitudes, it is necessary to control a composition effect caused by a change in the proportion of their elements. Otherwise, due to a composite effect, an increase in the number of well-educated women may superficially show different characteristics on birth cohorts in each round of repeated cross-sectional surveys. Taking these points into consideration, the inclusion of socio-economic variables in our model serves to control an effect caused by a compositional change in respondents.

As for the demographic variable, we employed the number of children a woman already had at the time of each survey. It is very likely that one's attitudes towards partnership and family differ according to one's family size. For instance, childlessness may have bearing upon a strong desire for self-fulfilment in life, whereas having many children may be linked to a conventional belief about the future prosperity of a family. In order to control the influence of these factors, we put the number of children a woman had as the level-1 explanatory variable of our analytical model. It should not, nevertheless, be forgotten that the demographic variable is not in a clear causal relation to the attitudinal variable. On the one hand, a strong preference for conventional family values may result in having many children. On the other hand, having many children may in itself cultivate a positive attitude to living in a large family. With the cross-sectional data, it is almost impossible to determine which of these two relations are the true causality of the attitude; therefore, our analysis limits itself to showing only a covariation between the two variables.

5.4 Descriptive Analysis of Attitudinal Change

The primary purpose of the present analysis is to investigate the influence of ages, periods and cohorts on attitudes towards partnership and family relations by using the HAPC method. Before that, this section attempts to compare and contrast attitudes between ages, periods and cohorts.

Graphs 5.4 and 5.5 display the relation between respondents' age and their attitudes, in each quinquennial round of the NSFJ. Graph 5.4 has the three opinion items (a) "Husband–wife segregation", (b) "Mother child-rearing" and (c) "Boys manly"; Graph 5.5 uses the other three items (d) "Marriage and children", (e) "Co-residence with parents" and (f) "Care for parents". In short, the former three opinion items are related to gender-relation attitudes, while the latter three have a bearing on inter-generational attitudes.

To begin with, let us look at the percentages of respondents who chose "strongly agree" and "agree" to opinion items (a) "Husband–wife segregation", (b) "Mother child-rearing" and (c) "Boys manly" in Graph 5.4. Two salient features should

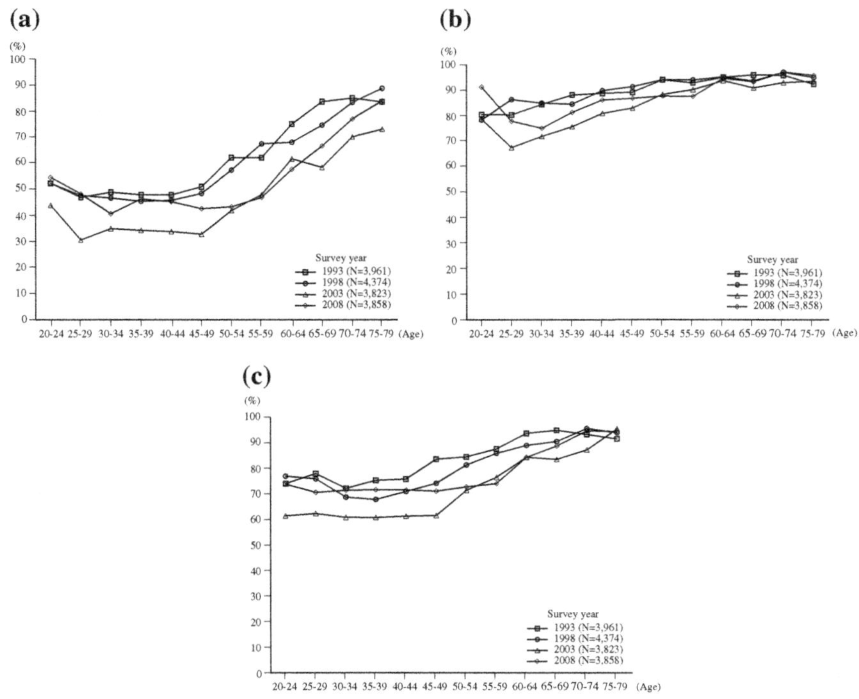

Graph 5.4 Percentage of women who support each opinion item by survey year (gender-relation attitude). **a** A husband should work outside and a wife should devote herself to doing housework after marriage. **b** It is better for a mother to devote herself to childrearing until her child reaches age three. **c** It is natural that boys are brought up manly and girls are brought up womanly

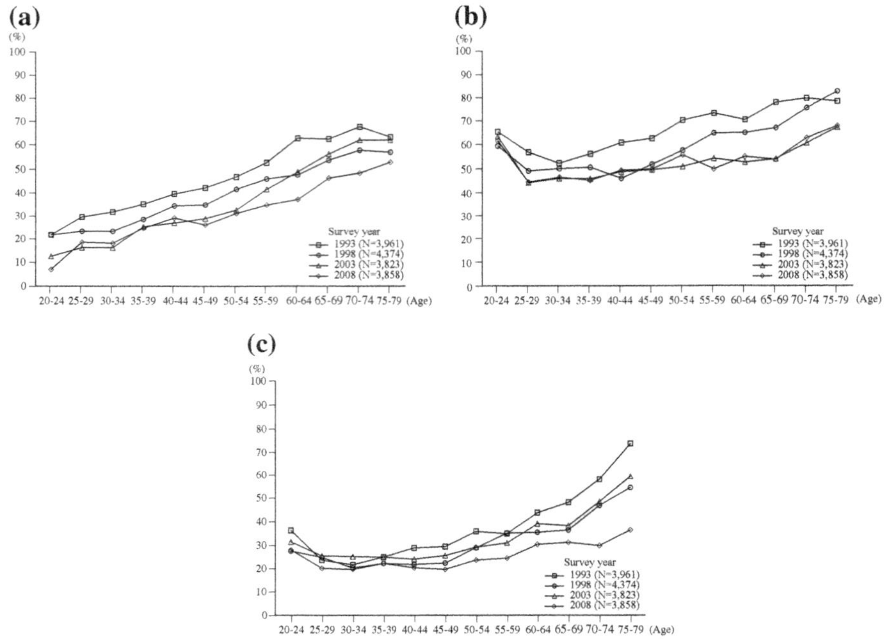

Graph 5.5 Percentage of women who support each opinion item by survey year (inter-generational relation attitude). **a** Marriage is socially accepted after a couple have children. **b** Children should live with their aged parents under the same roof. **c** It is children's duty to look after aged parents

be noted here. First, although percentages of women with a positive stance differ between three opinion items, a similar pattern is seen in the relation between age and attitudes. More specifically, the percentage of respondents who chose "strongly agree" or "agree" to each item stays relatively low until their 40 s and then gradually rises from their 50–70 s. For instance, when looking at the survey in 1998, the proportion of respondents supporting item (a) "Husband–wife segregation" remained around 50 % until the 45–49 age group and then steadily rose to 88.9 % at the 75–79 age group. This pattern caused by the ageing process is similar in all three items even if the absolute proportion of women with a positive stance differs between the opinion items. In the second place, attitudes towards gender relation fluctuate between the survey periods and do not change in a single direction. To be specific, the percentage of women having positive attitudes towards these three opinion items fell from the 1993 to the 2003 surveys, but increased in the survey of 2008. The periodical change of item (c) "Boys manly" is a case in point. In the 1993 survey, the proportion of respondents who strongly agreed or agreed with this opinion stood at over 70 % in all categories between ages 20 and 49. The percentage then gradually fell, reaching around 60 % in 2003, and then rose up again to over 70 % in 2008. This evidence suggests that value consciousness regarding traditional gender relation does not change in a fixed direction.

Now, let us turn to attitudes towards inter-generational relations. Graph 5.5 exhibits the percentages of respondents who chose "strongly agree" and "agree" with opinion item (d) "Marriage and children", (e) "Co-residence with parents" and (f) "Care for parents". As is the case with gender-relation values, the opinion items on inter-generational relations are supported more by older women than by younger women. Thus, the older those women become, the less individualistic their attitudes become. To exemplify, in the 1993 round of the NSFJ, the proportion of respondents who chose "strongly agree" or "agree" to opinion item (d) "Marriage and children" stood at less than 30 % until the 35–39 age group; the figure then rose to more than 60 % after the 60–64 age group. This right-hand upward relation between women's age and attitudes is commonly observed in these three items, although there is a difference in the absolute level supporting each opinion.

It is worth noting that, contrary to the case for gender-relation attitudes, inter-generational attitudes display a consistent downward trend across four rounds of the survey. More specifically, the percentage of women who strongly agree or agree with the opinions steadily declines from the 1993 to the 2008 survey. Opinion item (e) "Co-residence with parents" is a good case in point. In the 1993 survey, approximately 55 % of respondents in their 30 and 40 s thought that children should live with their aged parents under the same roof. The figure fell, however, to about 50 % in the 1998 survey, finally reaching around 45 % in the 2003 and 2008 surveys. It follows from this finding that, as time goes by, respondents less support a household composed of multiple generations and have more self (or couple)-centred attitudes.

At the same time, however, it should be borne in mind that these temporal changes in attitudes are not all attributable to period effects. This is because women who fall in a younger age group in an earlier survey will eventually be classified within older age groups in later survey. For instance, given that a considerable number of young women hold more negative attitudes towards conventional gender relations in an earlier survey, those with the same attitudes will, *ceteris paribus*, constitute a large proportion of older age groups in a later round of the survey. In other words, people with negative attitudes will move from younger to older categories over time. With this point in mind, it is too early to say from these findings whether traditional values wither, while individualistic attitudes become reinforced as time goes by. Thus, in order to scrutinize a trend in attitudinal changes in Japan, we will look at the relation between attitudes and birth cohorts from another angle.

Graphs 5.6 and 5.7 display variations in attitudes towards gender and inter-generational relations by birth cohort. Percentages in the graphs give us the proportion of respondents who chose "strongly agree" and "agree" for each opinion statement. For the sake of simplicity, we merged the pre-1924 birth cohort with the 1925–1929 cohort, and the post-1980 birth cohort with the 1975–1979 in the two graphs.

When it comes to gender-relation attitudes in Graph 5.6, a clear attitudinal shift can hardly be seen between birth cohorts. In other words, young cohorts do not

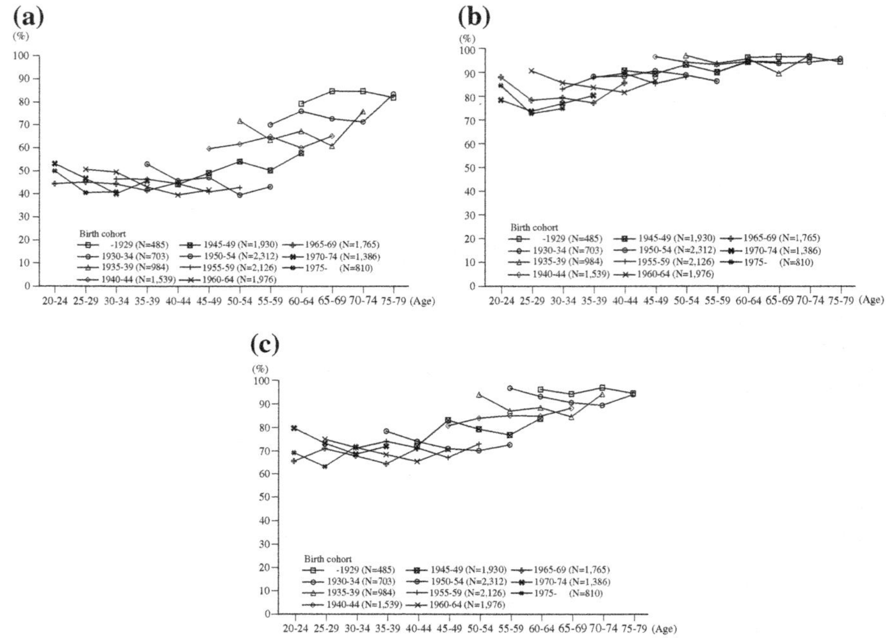

Graph 5.6 Percentage of women who support each opinion item by birth cohort (gender-relation attitude). **a** A husband should work outside and a wife should devote herself to doing housework after marriage. **b** It is better for a mother to devote herself to childrearing until her child reaches age three. **c** It is natural that boys are brought up manly and girls are brought up womanly

always hold more negative attitudes towards conventional gender relations than old cohorts. This feature is particularly conspicuous for cohorts born after 1950. Item (a) "Husband–wife segregation" is a good case in point. When looking at the period between ages 35 and 39, the 1950–1954 birth cohort yielded a highest percentage of 52.9, but the 1965–1969 cohort showed a lowest percentage of 41.5 %. Moreover, for the same age range in the 1970–1974 cohort, the figure reached 45.7 %, standing between the two cohorts. In the same vein, when women were from 30 to 34 years of age, 67.8 % of them agreed or strongly agreed with item (c) "Boys manly" in the 1965–1969 birth cohort. The percentage, however, stood at over 70 % in the 1960–1964 and post-1975 birth cohorts. We may argue from these findings that no consistent attitudinal change occurs among birth cohorts regarding gender-relation attitudes.

By contrast, where attitudes towards inter-generational relations are concerned, a somewhat clear transformation is observed across birth cohorts. More specifically, as seen from Graph 5.7, younger birth cohorts tend to hold a more individualistic attitude than older birth cohorts. To take a typical case, the percentage of women who agreed or strongly agreed with item (d) "Marriage and

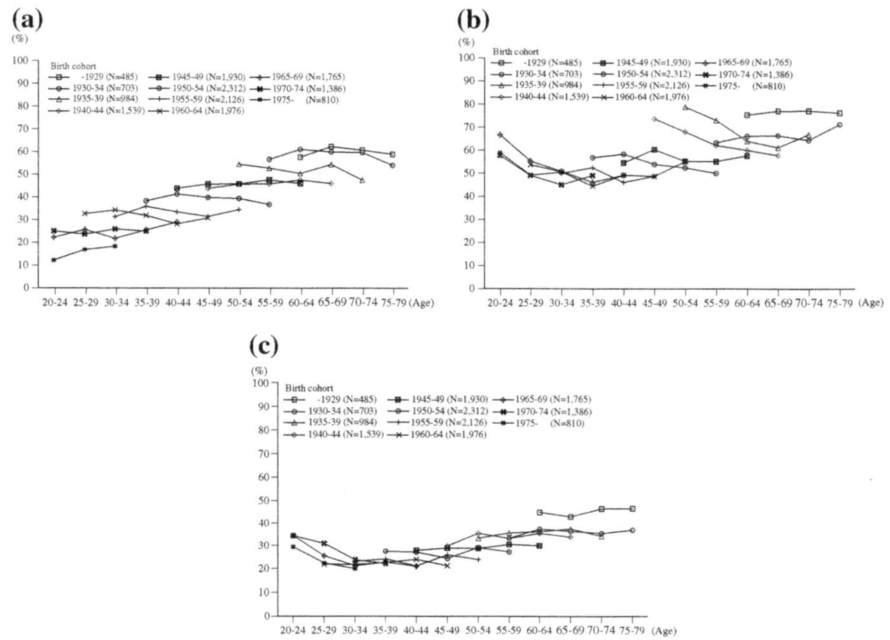

Graph 5.7 Percentage of women who support each opinion item by birth cohort (inter-generational relation attitude). **a** Marriage is socially accepted after a couple have children. **b** Children should live with their aged parents under the same roof. **c** It is children's duty to look after aged parents

children" remained stable at approximately 40 % in women from their late 30 s to their early 50 s within the 1950–1954 birth cohort. Yet, the percentage was lower, at about 35 %, in the same age range within the 1955–1959 cohort. The percentage of women who supported this opinion dropped even lower, to 30 %, in the 1960–1964 cohort. In short, the younger the birth cohort is, the less support this idea receives. By the same token, when looking at item (e) "Co-residence with parents", more than 60 % of women born before 1994 thought that children should live with their aged parents. As a result of loss in popularity, however, the percentage of women in support of this opinion decreased to about 50 % in birth cohorts from the 1950s and 1960s. This evidence suggests that, while the conventional inter-generational relations into which individuals are embedded become less influential cohort by cohort, individualistic lifestyles are gradually taking hold overall.

Of course, we should refrain from drawing a definite conclusion from the results of a descriptive analysis in this section. It is, nevertheless, safe to say that there is a difference in the patterns of ideational changes. To be specific, gender-relation attitudes do not show a consistent shift among birth cohorts and survey periods, while attitudes in inter-generational relations are steadily changing between cohorts and survey periods.

5.5 Results of the HACP Analysis of Attitudinal Change

In the previous section, we provided an overall picture of ideational changes in age, cohorts and periods. This section attempts to investigate the influence of age, cohorts and periods on attitudes towards gender and inter-generational relations by using HACP (Hierarchical Age-Cohort-Period) analysis. To begin with, we will examine gender-relation attitudes in Table 5.2. Model 1 of the table includes respondents' age and age squared, the number of children ever-born and educational levels as independent variables. As clearly seen in Model 1 of Table 5.2, both the linear and squared terms of age are statistically significant at the 1 % level. This means that the relation between the attitude and age is curvilinear. In addition, the sign of the coefficient is positive in the linear term, while it is negative in the squared term. It follows that attitudes to gender relations become rapidly conservative as the year of age increases.

When it comes down to the number of children, women who have no children hold a less traditional attitude to gender relations. In fact, compared with women who had two children, those without children yielded 0.247-point higher scores concerning gender-relation attitude. Yet, when women had more than or equal to a child, a significant coefficient was not observed. Hence, it follows that only childless women have a less conventional and more progressive attitude to gender relations.

As might be expected, the gender attitudinal score increases in tandem with a rise in women's educational level. Women whose formal education ended at a primary or junior high school yielded a 0.281-point lower attitudinal score than women with a high school diploma. In contrast, the attitudinal score was 1.140 points higher for women with a four-year university degree, while women with a two-year junior college diploma showed a 0.306-point higher score than women with solely a high school diploma. Moreover, a coefficient is statistically significant for all these variables. A higher educational qualification, therefore, leads to a less traditional attitude towards gender relations. These findings also allow us to infer that a compositional factor contributes to the overall change in gender attitudes. In other words, as more women enjoy a higher level of education, the proportion of women who have a more traditional attitude decreases. Accordingly, the overall level of opinion in support of traditional gender relations becomes low, *ceteris paribus*.

Model 2 of Table 5.2 was prepared to investigate period effects on attitudes. Its independent variables are composed of those in Model 1 and period variables. Interestingly, the coefficients of the model suggest that attitudes to gender relations experienced a backlash over the last 20 years. More specifically, since the coefficient increased from −0.147 in 1993 to 0.564 in 2003, it follows that gender-relation attitude became less traditional in this period. The figure, however, fell to 0.351 in 2008, indicating that the attitude had swung back towards the traditional. Where goodness of model fit is concerned, the log-likelihood ratio test between Models 1 and 2 was statistically significant at the 1 % level, the latter being a

Table 5.2 Results of HAPC analysis (gender relations)

Independent variables	Model 1	Model 2	Model 3	Model 4
Fixed effects	Coefficient	Coefficient	Coefficient	Coefficient
Constant	6.326***	6.472***	6.423***	6.508***
Age	0.020***	0.017***	0.018**	0.019**
Age squared	−0.001***	−0.001***	−0.001***	−0.001***
Education				
Primary or junior high school (high school)	−0.281**	−0.199**	−0.182***	
2-year junior college or vocational school	0.306**	0.249**	0.239***	
4-year university or higher	1.140***	1.064**	1.048***	
Spouse's annual income (less than 3,000,000 yen)				
3,000,000–6,000,000 yen				0.116***
Over 6,000,000 yen				0.192***
The number of children ever-born				
Childless	0.247***	0.198**	0.216**	0.329***
1 Child	0.070	0.033	0.045	0.088
(2 Children)				
3 Children	0.051	0.047	0.043	0.025
Over 3 Children	−0.092	−0.058	−0.063	−0.089
Random effects				
Cohort				
–1924			0.001	0.001
1925–1929			−0.127	−0.099
1930–1934			0.001	0.001
1935–1939			0.001	0.001
1940–1944			−0.150**	−0.161**
1945–1949			0.001	0.001
1950–1954			0.160**	0.190***
1955–1959			0.097**	0.180***
1960–1964			0.110**	0.180***
1965–1969			0.001	0.001
1970–1974			−0.066	−0.086
1975–1979			0.001	0.001
1980–			−0.236*	−0.268*
Period				
1993		−0.147***	−0.518***	−0.175***
1998		0.001	−0.364***	0.001
2003		0.564***	0.198***	0.631***
2008		0.351***	0.001	0.481***
Variance components	Variance	Variance	Variance	Variance
Individual	3.216**	3.141**	3.125**	3.219**

(continued)

Table 5.2 (continued)

Independent variables	Model 1	Model 2	Model 3	Model 4
Period		0.106*	0.109*	0.144*
Cohort			0.019***	0.029***
Log-likelihood	−32108.41	−31926.25	−31907.23	−32148.79
BIC	64323.31	63968.68	63,940.32	64,413.76
N	16,016	16,016	16,016	16,016

Parenthese denote a reference category
"Age" = respondent's age—15
* $p < 0.10$; ** $p < 0.05$; *** $p < 0.01$
Source The Japanese Generations and Gender Survey

better model than the former. Thus, it follows that period effects play a key role in women's attitudes towards gender relations.

In order to examine cohort effects, we included birth cohorts in Model 3 of Table 5.2. As far as the coefficients of birth cohorts show, no consistent trend is observed in terms of attitudes to gender relations. More specifically, the values of the coefficient stand at around naught before the 1935–1939 birth cohort. Thereafter, the figure remains relatively high between the 1950–1954 and 1960–1964 birth cohorts, but it decreases again after the 1965–1969 birth cohort. In addition, a statistically significant coefficient was seen only in the 1940–1944, 1950–1954, 1955–1959, 1960–64 and post-1980 birth cohorts. From these results, we can argue that, although attitudes to gender relations vary to some degree across birth cohorts, they do not change in a fixed direction.

As for goodness of model fit, the log-likelihood ratio test shows that Model 3 is significantly different from Model 2 at the 1 % level. In addition, the inter-class correlation of period effects (ρ_1) reached 0.33 in Model 3, while the inter-class correlation of cohort effects (ρ_2) was only 0.06. The former value is five times as great as the latter. Judging from these inter-class correlations, period effects are considerably greater than cohort effects on attitudes towards gender relations.

Instead of respondents' educational qualifications, spouses' (=husbands') income levels are placed in Model 4. The important point to note here is that the gender attitudinal score becomes higher as the level of income increases. To put it another way, the higher the income of the spouse, the less traditional the wife. In fact, compared with the "less than 3,000,000 yen" income group, attitudinal scores were 0.116 points higher in the "3,000,000–6,000,000 yen" group and 0.192 points higher in the "over 6,000,000 yen" group. As seen in Model 3, well-educated women tended to hold a more progressive attitude towards gender relations. In Model 4, it can be seen that the gender attitudes of women in the better-off class are less conventional than those in the worse-off class. Taking these findings into consideration, we may argue that higher socio-economic status leads to a progressive attitude towards gender relations.

Let us now turn to the examination of inter-generational attitudes. Table 5.3 displays the results of the HACP analysis concerning attitudes towards inter-generational relations. First of all, as in the case of gender attitude, the linear and squared terms of age are statistically significant at the 1 % level for the attitudinal scores for inter-generational relations. Moreover, the coefficient of the linear term shows a positive sign, while that of the squared term yields a negative sign. Hence, women's attitudes become rapidly more familialistic as they become old.

Second, the attitudinal scores increase as a woman's educational qualification rises. Indeed, compared with women with a high school diploma, those whose formal education ended at primary or junior high school yielded a −0.420-point lower score. By contrast, women who graduated from a two-year college or a vocational school showed a 0.105-point higher score, while women with a university degree had a 0.467-point higher score. In addition, all coefficients of the educational variable were statistically significant. This result indicates that better-educated women hold more individualistic attitudes than less-educated women.

As for the number of children ever-born, a saliently different relation is identified. In the case of gender-relation attitude, the number of children had hardly a clear effect on attitudinal scores. In contrast, this independent variable has a conspicuous impact on inter-generational attitude. Compared with women with two children, those without children produced a 0.183-point greater score. In the same vein, women with a single child also had a 0.083-point higher score. On the other hand, the coefficient for women having three children stood at −0.121, whereas the coefficient for women with more than three children reached fully −0.322. These results clearly show that the fewer children a woman has, the more individualistic she is.

When it comes down to period effects, unlike the case with gender-relation attitudes, a consistent trend is observed in Model 2 of Table 5.3. The coefficient of the period variable increased gradually from −0.293 in 1993 to 0.253 in 2008. Moreover, since the log-likelihood ratio test was significant at the 1 % level, Model 2 of Table 5.3 has a better goodness of fit than Model 1 in the same table. This evidence indicates that familialistic relations between generations are losing popularity as time goes by.

As for cohort effects, unlike the case with gender-relation attitudes, a clear relation is seen in Model 3 of Table 5.3. More specifically, although the attitudinal score has no change in the cohorts born before 1944, it starts to rise from the 1945–1949 cohort and reaches its peak at the 1960s cohort, thereafter decreasing to the post-1980 cohort. In fact, the coefficient of birth cohorts remained naught before the 1940–1944 cohort, but it stood at approximately 0.200 in cohorts born between 1950 and 1964. Furthermore, the coefficient reached −0.272 in the cohort born after 1980. It follows from this evidence that a value shift is clearly occurring across birth cohorts in terms of relations between generations. In addition, Model 3 of Table 5.3 showed a 1 % level significance with the log-likelihood ratio test, indicating that it has a better goodness of fit than Model 2 of the same table. Where an inter-class correlation is concerned, the period variable (ρ_1) stood at 0.16 in Model 3, whereas the cohort variable (ρ_2) reached 0.04. The former figure is

Table 5.3 Results of HAPC analysis (inter-generational relations)

Independent variables	Model 1	Model 2	Model 3	Model 4
Fixed effects	Coefficient	Coefficient	Coefficient	Coefficient
Constant	8.333***	8.443***	8.336***	8.265***
Age	0.021***	0.018***	0.024***	0.015***
Age squared	−0.001***	−0.001***	−0.001***	−0.001***
Education				
Primary or junior high school (high school)	−0.420***	−0.349***	−0.331***	
2-year junior college or vocational school	0.105**	0.060**	0.052**	
4-year university or higher	0.467***	0.405***	0.393***	
Spouse's annual income (less than 3,000,000 yen)				
3,000,000–6,000,000 yen				0.229***
Over 6,000,000 yen				0.396***
The number of children ever-born				
Childless	0.183***	0.151***	0.169***	0.229***
1 Child	0.083**	0.057**	0.071***	0.093***
(2 Children)				
3 Children	−0.121***	−0 119***	−0.120***	−0.128***
Over 3 Children	−0.322***	−0.292***	−0.287***	−0.309***
Random effects				
Cohort				
–1924			−0.094	−0.135
1925–1929			−0.118	−0.121
1930–1934			0.001	0.001
1935–1939			0.001	0.001
1940–1944			0.001	0.001
1945–1949			0.103**	0.110***
1950–1954			0.213***	0.226***
1955–1959			0.170***	0.165***
1960–1964			0.222***	0.249***
1965–1969			0.090***	0.050***
1970–1974			0.001	0.001
1975–1979			−0.001**	−0.003*
1980–			−0.272**	−0.345***
Period				
1993		−0.293***	−0.295***	−0.306***
1998		0.001	0.001	0.001
2003		0179***	0.185***	0.232***
2008		0.253***	0.274***	0.367***
Variance components	Variance	Variance	Variance	Variance
Individual	2.833**	2.792**	2.781***	2.788***

(continued)

Table 5.3 (continued)

Independent variables	Model 1	Model 2	Model 3	Model 4
Fixed effects	Coefficient	Coefficient	Coefficient	Coefficient
Period		0.044***	0.047**	0.065*
Cohort			0.012***	0.017***
Log-likelihood	−31,064.13	−30,956.38	−30,943.19	−30,967.42
BIC	62,234.75	62,028.94	62,012.24	62,051.02
N	16,016	16,016	16,016	16,016

Parenthese denote a reference category
"Age" = respondent's age—15
* $p < 0.10$; ** $p < 0.05$; *** $p < 0.01$
Source The Japanese Generations and Gender Survey

four times greater than the latter. This evidence means that the ratio of the two correlations (ρ_2 over ρ_1) is greater for inter-generational attitudes than for gender attitudes. It hence follows that the cohort effect has a stronger impact on attitudes towards inter-generational relations than on attitudes towards gender relations, whereas gender attitudes are more affected by the period effect. In other words, compared with gender relations, inter-generational relations experience a more salient value shift across birth cohorts.

Interestingly, the difference in coefficients between the educational categories becomes smaller in Model 3 than in Model 1 of Table 5.3. Indeed, although the difference between the "Primary or Junior High School" and the "4-year University or Higher" category stood at 0.887 points in Model 1, that decreased to 0.724 points in Model 3 of Table 5.3. This result allows us to infer that, when excluding the influence of period and cohort variables, the net effect of women's education is smaller than expected.

For the sake of examining the effect of economic status, Model 4 of Table 5.3 includes spouses' (husbands') incomes instead of women's educational levels. It is, at first glance, identifiable that the attitudinal scores increase as the income levels increase. Compared with women whose husbands earned less than 3,000,000 yen *per annum*, those in the "3,000,000–6,000,000 yen" group yielded a 0.229-point higher score. Moreover, when a husband's income reached over 6,000,000 yen, his wife's attitudinal score increased by 0.396 points. This evidence thus indicates that women in more affluent classes hold a relatively individualistic attitude. We should not, however, neglect the fact that the value of bayesian information criterion (BIC) is smaller for Model 3 in Table 5.3 than for Model 4 in the same table. This evidence means that the goodness of fit is greater for Model 3 than Model 4 of Table 5.3. Thus, we may argue that women's educational levels have a more explanatory power than spouses' incomes.

Finally, in order to understand the effects of age, cohorts and periods on attitudes graphically, we present predicted attitudinal scores in Graphs 5.8 and 5.9. All predicted scores were obtained by Model 3 in Tables 5.2 and 5.3, which had the best goodness of model fit with the smallest BIC. A thin black line with circles indicates estimated scores, while dotted lines on the upper and the lower side designate the corresponding 95 % confidence intervals of the estimated values. In addition, when age, cohort and period effects were estimated, all other independent variables were kept averaged.

Let us, first of all, look at attitudes towards gender relations with Graph 5.8. As has been already mentioned, the age effect on gender attitudes is curvilinear over the life course (see the top panel of Graph 5.8). It is conspicuously clear that the predicted score reaches its peak around age 30 and falls with increasing acceleration after around age 40. As for the cohort effect, no consistent trend was identified across birth cohorts, even in the graphical presentation (see the middle panel of Graph 5.8). Although a rise in the predicted value occurs in cohorts between 1950 and 1964, there is, as a whole, no clear trend in attitudes towards gender relations. On the other hand, the period effect shows an interesting shift (see the bottom panel of Graph 5.8). As far as the predicted scores show, conventional gender relation becomes less popular until 2003, but thereafter regains its popularity.

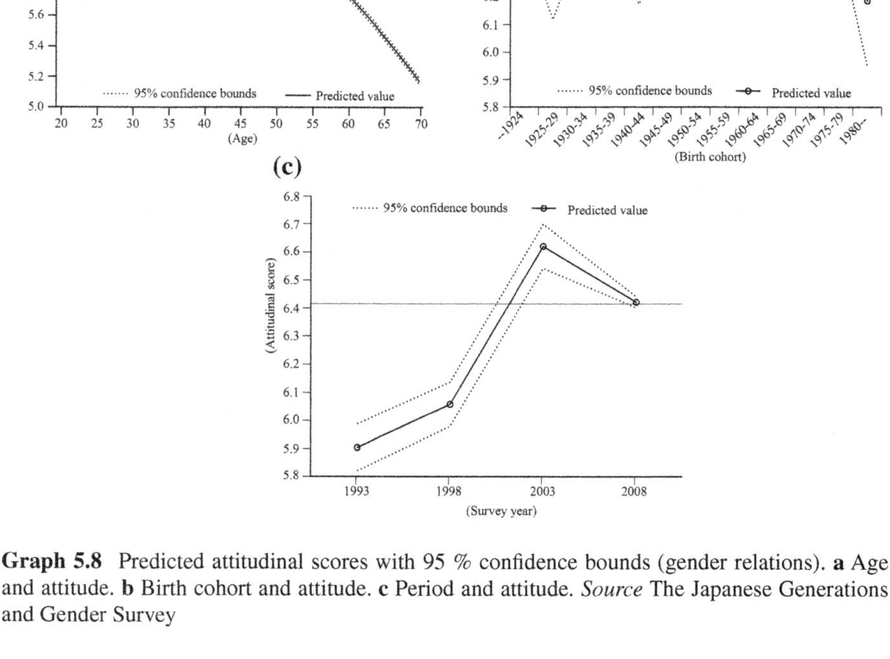

Graph 5.8 Predicted attitudinal scores with 95 % confidence bounds (gender relations). **a** Age and attitude. **b** Birth cohort and attitude. **c** Period and attitude. *Source* The Japanese Generations and Gender Survey

As in the case of gender attitude, inter-generational attitude also shows a curvilinear relation to women's age (see the top panel of Graph 5.9). Although the highest score shifts to a slightly older age in inter-generational attitude, the overall shape of the predicted line is almost the same in both sets of attitudinal scores. It follows, hence, that women rapidly shift towards less individualistic attitudes post-middle age. There is also a considerable difference between cohorts' attitudes to inter-generational and gender relations (see the middle panel of Graph 5.9). Although the predicted attitudinal score of inter-generational relations tends to increase until the 1960–1964 birth cohort, this trend reverses and decreases for women born after those years. Thus, we may argue that women's attitudes became individualistic up to birth cohorts born in the early 1960, after which their attitudes made a *volte face* and shifted towards more familialistic opinions again. The period effect, unlike the case with gender-relation attitudes, displays a consistent shift towards individualistic attitudes (see the bottom panel of Graph 5.9). In fact, the predicted score of inter-generational relations has a steady temporal rise, which indicates that an individualistic attitude towards inter-generational relations

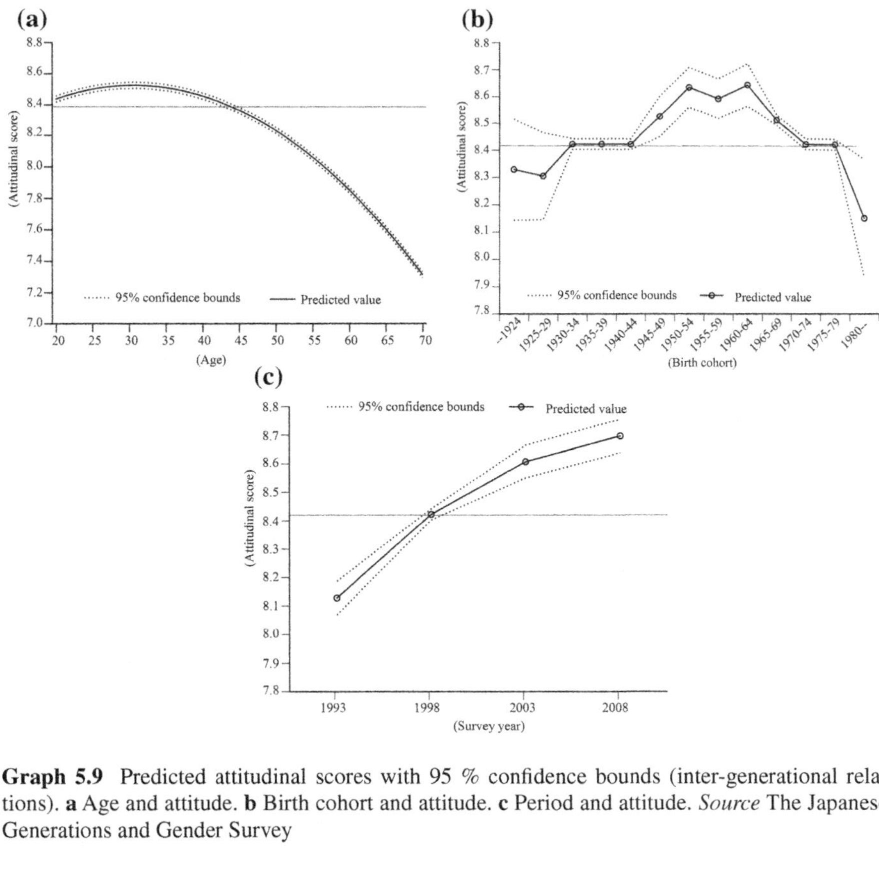

Graph 5.9 Predicted attitudinal scores with 95 % confidence bounds (inter-generational relations). **a** Age and attitude. **b** Birth cohort and attitude. **c** Period and attitude. *Source* The Japanese Generations and Gender Survey

is becoming more supported as time goes by. We lack definite information on the causes of this temporal change, but it is certain that familialistic ideas and values are gradually losing popularity.

5.6 Conclusion

The primary purpose of this chapter was to investigate an ideational transformation in Japan from a long perspective. In concrete terms, the effects of age, cohorts and periods on attitudes were examined by the HACP analysis in the chapter. Furthermore, as our two indicators of ideational shift, we employed attitudes towards gender and inter-generational relations.

The results of the analysis in the present chapter show, first of all, that women's age has a curvilinear relation to their attitudes. While traditional gender and inter-generational relations were supported the least by women around age 30, they both rapidly regained their popularity with women after age 40. Hence, judging from the results of our HACP analysis, we may argue that values and attitudes are not fixed, but malleable through one's life course. Second, we were able to identify that these two attitudinal indicators have a different period effect. The influence of individualistic attitudes towards inter-generational relations has been steadily strengthening over more recent periods, while the influence of traditional gender attitudes, which was once weakening, is becoming stronger again. These findings suggest that more importance is being attached to one's own individual life over family life in Japan. In this sense, we may argue that self-fulfilment or self-realization is commanding a more influential place in people's lives as time goes by. Third, our analysis found that the relation between birth cohorts and attitudes differs depending on the indicator: although no clear attitudinal shift could be identified across cohorts in terms of gender relations, attitudes towards inter-generational relations changed clearly across birth cohorts. More specifically, individualistic attitudes increasingly gained in force until the 1960–1964 birth cohort, afterwards which they relaxed. These results allow us to infer that the change in marriage and fertility behaviour seen in Japan from the 1970s until the 1990s is related to a value shift. As mentioned before, this behavioural shift coincided with the period when cohorts born from the 1950s to the early 1960s reached adulthood. Given that this generation has a more individualistic attitude, it seems likely that they attached a higher priority to self-fulfilment than to marriage and child-bearing. Thus, this ideational change can be regarded as one of the causes which prevailed the postponement of marriage and brought about the decline of fertility in Japan from the 1970s until the 1990s. We must not, however, overlook the fact that Japanese marriage and fertility behaviour have continued to shift along the same lines well into the 2000s. As seen in the results of our analysis, birth cohorts who entered into adulthood in the twenty-first century show a less individualistic attitude than previous birth cohorts. Birth cohorts after the early 1970s who entered adulthood after the bubble economy are not relatively self-centred, but they tend to be reluctant to marry and have children. Taking this point into consideration, it is difficult to explain more recent changes in Japanese marriage and fertility patterns only by the ideational theory. In other words, it may be concluded that a superficially continuous demographic phenomenon is caused by different underlying factors.

References

Aassve, A., Sironi, M., & Bassi, V. (2013). Explaining attitudes towards demographic behaviour. *European Sociological Review, 29*, 316–333.

Ariès, P. (1980). Two successive motivations for the declining birth rate in the west. *Population and Development Review, 6*, 645–650.

Bauman, Z. (2000). *Liquid modernity*. Cambridge: Polity Press.

Beck, U., Giddens, A., & Lash, S. (1994). *Reflexive modernization: Politics, tradition and aesthetics in the modern social order*. Cambridge: Polity Press.

Bell, D. (1976). *The cultural contradictions of capitalism*. New York: Basic Books.

Clarke, H. D., Kornberg, A., McIntyre, C., Bauer-Kaase, P., & Kaase, M. (1999). The effect of economic priorities on the measurement of value change: New experimental evidence. *The American Political Science Review, 93*, 637–647.

Durkheim, É. (1956). *Education and sociology*. Glencoe: Free Press.

Esping-Andersen, G. (1990). *The three worlds of welfare capitalism*. Cambridge: Polity Press.

Esping-Andersen, G. (1999). *Social foundations of postindustrial economies*. Oxford: Oxford University Press.

Ferarra, M. (1996). The 'southern model' of welfare in social Europe. *Journal of European Social Policy, 6*, 17–37.

Fienberg, S. E., & Mason, W. M. (1985). Specification and Implementation of age, period and cohort models. In W. M. Mason & S. E. Fienberg (Eds.), *Cohort Analysis in Social Research: Beyond the Identification Problem* (pp. 45–88). New York: Springer.

Fukuda, N. (2003). Comparing family-friendly policies in Japan and Europe: Are we in the same or in a different league? *Journal of Population and Social Security, 1*, 31–45.

Gauthier, A. H. (1996). *The state and the family*. Oxford: Clarendon Press.

Gauthier, A. H., & Hatzius, J. (1997). Family benefits and fertility: An econometric analysis. *Population Studies, 51*, 295–306.

Gauthier, A. H., & Philipov, D. (2008). Can policies enhance fertility in europe? *Vienna Yearbook of Population Research, 2008*, 1–16.

Glenn, N. D. (1989). A caution about mechanical solutions to the identification problem in cohort analysis: comment on Sasaki and Suzuki. *American Journal of Sociology, 95*, 754–761.

Glenn, N. D. (2003). Distinguishing age, period, and cohort effects. In J. T. Mortimer & M. J. Shanahan (Eds.), *Handbook of the life course* (pp. 465–76). New York: Kluwer Academic/Plenum Publishers.

Goodman, R., & Peng, I. (1996). The east asian welfare states. In G. Espin-Andersen (Ed.), *Welfare states in transition: National adaptations in global economies* (pp. 192–224). London: Sage.

Gornick, J. C., Meyers, M., & Ross, K. (1997). Supporting the employment of mothers: Policy variation across fourteen welfare states. *Journal of European Social Policy, 7*, 45–70.

Haller, M. (2002). Theory and method in the comparative study of values: Critique and alternative to Inglehart. *European Sociological Review, 18*, 139–158.

Halman, L., Inglehart, R., Díez-Medrano, J., Luijkx, R., Morena, A., & Basáñez, M. (Eds.). (2008). *Changing values and beliefs in 85 countries: Trends from the values surveys from 1981 to 2004*. Leiden: Brill.

Hauser, R. M. (1970). Context and consex: A cautionary tale. *American Journal of Sociology, 75*, 645–664.
Hobcraft, J, Menken J, & Preston, S. (1985). Age, period, and cohort effects in demography: A review. In W. M. Mason & S. E. Fienberg (Eds.) *Cohort Analysis in Social Research: Beyond the Identification Problem* (pp. 89–135). New York: Springer.
Inglehart, R. (1977). *The silent revolution: Changing values and political styles among western publics*. Princeton: Princeton University Press.
Inglehart, R. (1990). *Culture shift in advanced industrial society*. Princeton: Princeton University Press.
Inglehart, R. (1995). Changing values, economic development and political change. *International Social Science Journal, 47*, 379–403.
Inglehart, R. (1997). *Modernization and postmodernization: cultural, economic, and political change in 43 societies*. Princeton: Princeton University Press.
Inglehart, R. (Ed.). (2003). *Human values and social change: Findings from the values surveys*. Leiden: Brill.
Inglehart, R., & Baker, W. E. (2000). Modernization, cultural change, and the persistence of traditional values. *American Sociological Review, 65*, 19–51.
Inglehart, R., & Basañez, M. (Eds.). (2010). *Changing human beliefs and values, 1981–2007: A cross-cultural sourcebook based on the world values surveys and european values studies*. D.F., Siglo Veintiuno Editores: México.
Inglehart, R., & Welzel, C. (2005). *Modernization, cultural change, and democracy: The human development sequence*. Cambridge: Cambridge University Press.
Jagodzinski, W. (1983). Materialism in Japan reconsidered: Toward a synthesis of generational and life-cycle explanations. *The American Political Science Review, 77*, 887–894.
Lesthaeghe, R. (1983). A century of demographic and cultural change in Western Europe. *Population and Development Review, 9*, 411–436.
Lewis, J. (1992). Gender and the development of Welfare Regimes. *Journal of European Social Policy, 2*, 159–173.
Maslow, A. H. (1970). *Motivation and personality*. New York: Harper & Row.
Mason, W. M., & Fienberg, S. E. (Eds.). (1985). *Cohort analysis in social research: Beyond the identification problem*. New York: Springer.
Mason, K. O., Mason, W. M., Winsborough, H. H., & Kenneth Poole, W. (1973). Some methodological issues in cohort analysis of archival data. *American Sociological Review, 38*, 242–258.
Merton, R. K. (1968). *Social theory and social structure*. New York: Free Press.
Newson, L., & Richerson, P. J. (2009). Why do people become modern? A darwinian explanation. *Population and Development Review, 35*, 117–158.
Parsons, T., & Bales, R. F. (Eds.). (1955). *Family, socialization and interaction process*. New York: Free Press.
Raudenbush, S. W., & Bryk, A. S. (2002). *Hierarchical linear models: Applications and data analysis methods*. Thousand Oaks: Sage Publications.
Sainsbury, D. (1994). Women's and men's social rights: Gendering dimensions of welfare states. In D. Sainsbury (Ed.), *Gendering welfare states* (pp. 150–69). London: SAGE Publications.
Salles, A. (2006). The effects of family policy in the former GDR on nuptiality and births outside marriage. *Population (English Edition), 61*, 141–151.
Sasaki, M., & Suzuki, T. (1987). Changes in religious commitment in the United States, Holland, and Japan. *American Journal of Sociology, 92*(5), 1055–1076.
Siaroff, A. (1994). Work, welfare and gender equality: A new typology. In D. Sainsbury (Ed.), *Gendering welfare states* (pp. 82–100). London: SAGE Publications.
Thévenon, O. (2011). Family policies in OECD countries: A comparative analysis. *Population and Development Review, 37*, 57–87.
Tranter, B., & Western, M. (2003). Postmaterial values and age: The case of Australia. *Australian Journal of Political Science, 38*, 239–257.

Wrigley, E. A. (1978). Fertility strategy for the individual and the group. In C. Tilly (Ed.), *Historical studies of changing fertility* (pp. 135–154). Princeton: Princeton University Press.
Yang, Y. (2008). Social inequalities in happiness in the United States, 1972 to 2004: An age-period-cohort analysis. *American Sociological Review, 73*, 204–226.
Yang, Y., & Land, K. C. (2006). A mixed models approach to the age-period-cohort analysis of repeated cross-section surveys, with an application to data on trends in verbal test scores. *Sociological Methodology, 36*, 75–97.
Yang, Y., & Land, K. C. (2008). Age-period-cohort analysis of repeated cross-section surveys: Fixed or random effects? *Sociological Methods & Research, 36*, 297–326.
Yang, Y., & Land, K. C. (2013). *Age-period-cohort analysis: New models, methods, and empirical applications*. Boca Raton: CRC Press.

Chapter 6
Conclusion

6.1 Introduction

As stated in Chap. 1, this book focuses on the two main themes. The first purpose is to examine the influence of economic and ideational factors on Japanese marriage and fertility behaviour. As discussed in Chap. 2, from the viewpoint of social action theory, economic and ideational frameworks can be regarded as the most appropriate tools for the analysis of marriage and childbearing patterns. At the same time, indelibly engraved in both frameworks are the methodological and epistemological characteristics of human behaviour inherent in these theories. Thus, it was crucial to examine and evaluate the relevance and suitability of these theoretical frameworks in the analysis of marriage and fertility patterns in contemporary Japan. The second purpose of this book is to investigate a historical change in attitudes towards partnership and family in Japan. While the relation between economic change and demographic behaviour attracted much research attention in Japan, the transformation in attitudes towards partnership and family had yet to receive any thorough examination from a historical perspective. However, in order to understand a temporal change in marriage and fertility patterns, it is essential to investigate this shift in values and attitudes over a long range of time. Hence, this book dealt with a historical change in attitudes towards gender and inter-generational relations.

Following these research interests, we theoretically and empirically examined marriage and fertility behaviour in the previous chapters by using data from panel and repeated cross-sectional surveys. In this final chapter, we will first summarize the main arguments and empirical findings presented in the previous chapters. Thereafter, we will conclude this book by discussing the implications of this study for marriage and fertility behaviour.

N. Fukuda, *Marriage and Fertility Behaviour in Japan*,
DOI 10.1007/978-981-10-0294-6_6

6.2 Rationality and Demographic Behaviour

As a starting point of this book, we considered two theoretical frameworks regarding marriage and fertility behaviour in developed countries: the economic theory and the ideational theory.

Since almost all human beings form marital unions and build families within societies, these behaviours can be seen as social actions. In other words, marriage and fertility behaviour are not performed in a social vacuum. Rather, the characteristics of the society in which individuals live are strongly reflected in their patterns of partnership formation and family building. Taking this position, it becomes indispensable to examine marriage and childbearing behaviour from a viewpoint of social action. Since it is claimed in the economic and ideational theories that marriage and fertility behaviour are actions taken in human society, their analytical frameworks can be based on the theory of social action.

As discussed in Chap. 2 in detail, however, the economic and the ideational theories posit that the mechanisms of marriage and fertility behaviour are understood from entirely different perspectives. The economic theory interprets marriage and childbirth behaviour from a material and objective point of view, while the ideational theory accounts for these behaviours from a psychological and motivational standpoint. This difference between the two theories originates in their methodological and epistemological models of a human action. In the economic model, the purpose of a human action is to optimally allocate limited social resources such as wages and time in order to maximize satisfaction. Furthermore, it is postulated that the structure of satisfaction is determined by stable and exogenously given preferences. In this model, therefore, the attainment of a goal with the minimum cost occupies a central position in explaining the choice of an action. In contrast, the ideational theory postulates a preference-centred heuristic model of human behaviour. Preference is formulated by subjective meanings and discursive interpretations produced by individual beliefs and values. These beliefs and values consequently work in an individual to define desirable conduct. To put it another way, in the ideational model, one behaves in the way that accords with one's beliefs and values.

Although the two theories have different behavioural models and analytical frameworks with reference to marriage and childbearing behaviour, the methodological and epistemological distance between the two is not so great as is thought. Rather, the behavioural models of the two theories are reinterpreted in an integrated way from the viewpoint of rational choice theory. This can be clearly understood by utilizing the two types of rational action proposed by Weber (1978a, b, 2002). The first of these types is an instrumental rational action, which is taken by the actor to attain a predetermined goal at minimal expense. As mentioned before, a choice in human action is made, according to the economic theory, to maximize a fixed preference with the minimum cost. In this respect, the behavioural model for the economic theory can be seen to reflect Weber's formulation of instrumental rational action. Weber's second type of action is a value-rational action, which is motivated, regardless of the possible costs, by an actor's own beliefs and values. The ideational theory holds that marriage and fertility patterns are determined not by economic cost–benefit calculation, but by human beliefs and values. In view of that, the behavioural model of this theory can be seen in terms of value-rational action. Thus, looking from a viewpoint of rationality, the behavioural models of the two theories can be included under the rubric of rational conduct. In other words, what makes a distinction between the two theories is the type of rationality postulated.

It is, however, difficult to determine theoretically which of the two types of rational action is more relevant in the interpretation of marriage and childbearing behaviour in a specific developed society. After all, institutional settings formally or informally give structural incentives and disincentives to choices in human action (North 1990, 2005). Marriage and fertility patterns may be determined by instrumental rationality in one institutional environment, while they may be guided by value-rationality in another institutional environment. In other words, the impact of economic and ideational factors will vary from one country to another. Hence, without empirical analysis, it is impossible to determine the factors that play a key role in marriage and fertility patterns in Japan. Undoubtedly, carrying out an empirical analysis of marriage and childbearing patterns is the best way to clarify the mechanism of Japanese demographic behaviour. This is the central aim of this study.

6.3 Marriage Behaviour in Contemporary Japan

Several interesting features of Japanese marriage behaviour were revealed in the analysis of the panel survey's data in Chap. 3. First of all, economic factors had an important bearing on marriage patterns in Japan. More specifically, men and women with a large income tended to get married with a greater probability than those with a lower level of income. Furthermore, people engaged in a professional or a managerial job were more likely to enter into marriage. As mentioned before, the economic theory places great importance on material costs and benefits in the decision-making of marriage behaviour. Admittedly, our findings endorse the importance of economic calculations, but the influence of female earning capability on marriage does not entirely support the framework of the economic theory. To be specific, according to Becker's economic approach, a great gap in earning capability between men and women enhances a willingness to get married, while economic parity discourages marriage. Yet, this is not always the case in Japan. Rather, not only men's but also women's greater earning capacity encouraged marriage. This result suggests that women's greater economic power increases their willingness to marry by brightening their prospects in life after marriage. In addition, when comparing the influence of economic factors on men and women in their attitudes towards partnership and family, striking differences were seen. Men with a very high income tended to have more conservative attitudes, whereas high-salaried women's attitudes were more progressive. It follows that an increase in economic power appears to produce different attitudes when experienced by women as compared to men.

Second, ideational factors, at the same time, affected marriage behaviour in Japan, although their effects were not as strong as those of economic factors. Men with more progressive and individualistic attitudes tended to remain single. Likewise, women were less willing to enter into marriage as women's progressive and individualistic attitudes became strong. According to the ideational theory, a change in partnership relation originates in a value shift caused by affluence and security in developed countries. The results of our analysis are theoretically in accordance with this explanation. Yet, judging from the medium-level explanatory power of attitudinal variables, ideational factors have, in effect, a limited impact on Japanese marriage behaviour.

6.4 Fertility Behaviour in Contemporary Japan

As in the case of marriage behaviour, we examined in Chap. 4 the influence of economic and ideational factors on Japanese fertility behaviour with data from panel surveys.

The findings of this analysis revealed, first of all, that neither husbands' nor wives' incomes affected fertility behaviour significantly. In other words, the levels of their earning capabilities are not related to their decision on whether to have children. The economic theory holds that parents' income levels exercise an influence on fertility patterns by the amount of costs and benefits entailed by having children. Yet, our results do not support this theoretical presumption. Rather, they suggest that such economic factors play no substantial role in determining fertility patterns. Thus, we may argue that the framework of economic theory is not of great relevance when seeking explanations for Japanese fertility behaviour. In addition, the results of our analysis revealed that couples' incomes affect their attitudes towards partnership and family relations. Higher-salaried wives were relatively progressive, whereas husbands with a medium-level income had more conservative attitudes. In other words, economic status affected the cognitive framing (Goffman 1986) of partnership and family relations, although there was a gender difference in the influence of earning power.

Second, female employment status had a salient influence on fertility behaviour. Wives who were engaged in full-time employment tended to have fewer children. As mentioned above, since wives' incomes did not influence their childbearing patterns, it is reasonable to conclude that that the effects of female employment status may be interpreted not as signifiers of the level of opportunity costs entailed by childbirth and childrearing, but as signifiers of compatibility between employment and childrearing. This being the case, it follows that difficulty in harmonizing employment and family roles brings about a reluctance to have children. Taking this point into consideration, we may argue that the conflict between family and employment plays a crucial role in determining fertility patterns in Japan.

Third, our analysis found that ideational factors have an impact on fertility behaviour. Husbands and wives with progressive and individualistic attitudes had a lower probability of having a child than those with traditional and familialistic attitudes. The ideational theory attributes recent demographic changes in developed countries to a transformation in value-orientations. The results of our study are in accord with this explanation of the ideational theory. It is therefore safe to say that Japanese fertility behaviour is affected by ideational factors, although their influence is not so great. Interestingly, the influence of ideational factors tended to be strong for wives in full-time employment, but weak for those who were not employed. Taking this evidence into consideration, we may argue that female economic autonomy affects the relation between ideational factors and fertility behaviour.

6.5 Social Change and a Value Shift

Despite a difference in the extent of influence, we found in the previous two chapters that nuptial and fertility behaviour were affected by individual values and attitudes. At the same time, however, it should not be forgotten that patterns of marriage and fertility have been changing in Japan over the couple of decades. As discussed before, a value shift is regarded as a long-lasting and continuous process (Ariès 1980; Lesthaeghe 1983). Thus, in order to fully understand the relation between ideational and demographic patterns, attitudinal changes in Japan need to be examined from a long-range temporal perspective. Taking this point into consideration, in Chap. 5, we investigated whether attitudes towards partnership and family relations differ between ages, birth cohorts, and temporal periods in Japan by using the data of repeated cross-sectional surveys.

Several interesting findings were obtained from the analysis of Chap. 5. First, women's age had a curvilinear relation to their attitudes. Traditional gender and inter-generational relations were unpopular until around age 30, but showed a dramatic increase in popularity after age 40. To put it another way, while attitudes are progressive and self-oriented in early adulthood, they become more traditional and less individualistic in one's later years. Thus, it is safe to say that values and attitudes are not fixed throughout life.

Second, we see differences in temporal shift when examining attitudes towards traditional gender and inter-generational relations. Individualistic features clearly manifested themselves in inter-generational relations in more recent periods, whereas a consistent historical trend towards transformation was barely perceptible in the conventional values of gender relations. In short, there is a marked difference between the extent of period effects in the traditional and individualistic spheres of value-orientation in Japan. According to the ideational theory, due to an increase in affluence and security in society, the weakening of traditional values occurs in tandem with the strengthening of individualism. Yet, as far as the results of our analysis show, this is not the case in Japan. Rather, while an individualistic lifestyle is commanding a steadily increasing place in people's lives in more recent years, the influence of traditional gender values and norms is not diminishing monotonically.

Third, as for the relation between birth cohorts and attitudes, although no clear attitudinal shift was identified across cohorts regarding gender relations, attitudes towards inter-generational relations changed clearly across birth cohorts. More specifically, although birth cohorts between 1950 and 1964 became slightly less conventional, no discernable change was, as a whole, observed in an attachment to the traditional values of gender relations. In contrast, individualistic attitudes increasingly prevailed until the 1960–1964 birth cohorts, afterwards which they relaxed. Since cohorts born from the 1950s to the early 1960s reached adulthood between the 1970s and the 1990s, it seems likely that a change in the marriage and childbearing patterns of these years is related to the spread of individualistic attitudes among the birth cohorts. It must be noted, however, that despite the fact that Japanese marriage and fertility behaviour continued to change after the 2000s, birth cohorts with a less individualistic attitude entered into adulthood in this period exhibited a less individualistic attitude. We may interpret from these findings that more recent marriage and fertility patterns are less related to ideational changes.

6.6 Implications for the Economic Theory of Family Formation

As summarized above, the detailed analysis of Japanese marriage and fertility behaviour in this study furnished many interesting results for scholars. These findings naturally lead us to further consideration of the theories of marriage and fertility behaviour while they shed fresh light on the influence of economic and ideational factors on demographic behaviour in Japan. In this section, we will explore the implications of our findings on the economic theory.

As argued in Chap. 2 in detail, the economic theory—either the New Home Economic Theory or the Easterlin Theory—points the focus of demographic behaviour on material cost–benefit calculations. In short, one behaves in such a way as to maximize exogenously given utility (satisfaction) at the minimum cost. This is a key theorem underpinning the decision-making process of marriage and fertility behaviour in the economic theory. From a methodological viewpoint, this model of human behaviour is guided and directed by instrumental or economic rationality. For example, if forming a marital union will bring more satisfaction to the parties from the viewpoint of instrumental rationality, people will get married. Otherwise, they will remain single. Likewise, if the arrival of a newborn baby increases a couple's utility with a cost–benefit calculation, they will decide to have children. Of course, the amount of expenses one can afford for marriage and childrearing and the amount of satisfactions one can form gain marital partnership and parenthood differ in relation to one's earning power and economic status. Yet, the certain thing is that economic factors are presumed to play a crucial role in determining marriage and fertility patterns. This is a fundamental framework of the economic theory.

Yet, the results of our analysis are not perfectly in accordance with this framework. Admittedly, economic factors played a key role in marriage behaviour in Japan. Greater economic power encouraged men and women to marry. This evidence clearly indicates that instrumental or economic rationality commands a dominant position in a decision-making on marriage. However, neither husband's nor wives' incomes showed any significant bearing on fertility patterns. Japanese couples gave birth to children, regardless of their income levels. In this regard, instrumental or economic rationality does not have a substantial influence on fertility behaviour. In other words, it may be safe to that the economic theory is not always a suitable framework from with which to explain of Japanese fertility patterns.

At the same time, these findings of our analysis allow us to infer that there are various connections between economic power and demographic behaviour. More specifically, marriage and fertility behaviour have been separately formulated in the orthodox framework of the economic theory. This means that one's decision-making process in marital union formation is not directly linked to that of family building. Yet, judging from the results of our analysis, the entry to marriage tends to be explicitly or implicitly linked to having children in Japan. Thus, it would be better to analyse jointly the two demographic events of Japanese people. Indeed, as shown in Chap. 4, the proportion of out-of-wedlock births over all births is much lower in Japan than in other developed countries. This implies that marriage is still a dominant institution for procreation in Japan. To put it the other way round, when Japanese people make a decision on marriage, they may consider the cost–benefit of having children in married life as well. In short, the economic cost–benefit calculation on married life and child rearing may already be made at the time of decision-making on marriage. This being the case, it seems likely that economic factors have a very negligible impact on fertility behaviour. In particular, where a society has institutional settings supporting a "strong family" system, parents, especially mothers, have a greater responsibility for children's well being (Zuanna and Micheli 2004). In such a society, it is possible that a decision on whether to marry encompasses costs and benefits entailed in childrearing after marriage. Moreover, it should be recalled here that women's compatibility vis à vis employment and childcare played a crucial role in Japanese fertility patterns. These characteristics may be hallmarks of "strong family". Putting aside any judgement as to whether a Japanese family might be a strong family, the results of this study suggest that a theoretical framework of joint decision-making (or life-course decision-making) in marriage and fertility is useful when elaborating on the economic theory of fertility and marriage behaviour. In other words, the economic approach may need a framework to analyse the whole range of life course in an integrated way.

6.7 Implications for the Ideational Theory of Family Formation

Now let us turn to implications for the ideational theory. As shown before, we investigated the influence of ideational factors on Japanese marriage and fertility behaviour. Findings from our analysis also bear implications for elaborating the ideational theory further.

To begin with, although it was observed that ideational factors affect marriage and fertility behaviour in this study, the extent of their influence was relatively minor. Admittedly, people with progressive and individualistic attitudes had a lower probability of getting married or giving birth to children than those with conventional and family-centred attitudes. Yet, as far as the estimated coefficients of attitudinal variables shows, the patterns of marriage and childbearing are not so drastically affected by beliefs and values. As expressed in Chap. 2, the ideational theory holds that marriage and childbearing behaviour are guided and motivated by the beliefs and values an actor holds. Thus, these actions are, regardless of the possible costs, put into practice as long as it is valuable and desirable to an actor. More specifically, if forming a marital union or giving birth to children agree with one's values and beliefs, one will most likely chose to get married and have children. Otherwise, one will remain single and childless. The findings of this study, however, suggest that one's value-orientations do not play such a decisive role in marriage and fertility behaviour in Japan. In other words, value-rationality does not affect human conduct so deeply as is theoretically presumed.

This evidence takes us to a reconsideration of the relation between ideational factors and demographic behaviour. According to a behavioural model of the ideational theory, since one's conduct is guided and directed by one's values and beliefs, one would propose to take actions harmonizing with these ideas. Such actions eventually would provide psychological satisfaction to the actor. This is the central framework of value-rational action. Thus, one could assume that actions that do not to harmonize with one's values and beliefs will hardly be performed by the actor. However, this assumption does not appear to hold true in the case of Japan. As mentioned before, even when people have progressive and individualistic attitudes, their disinclination towards marrying and having children tends to be considerably suppressed. Thus, despite the fact that progressive and individualistic values and ideas are largely found to be ideologically attractive in Japan, this attraction does not reach the point where marriage formation and family building are rejected immediately. Rather, in order to avoid perceived obstacles and anticipated impediments and minimize the psychological cost entailed by deviation from a conventional behaviour, Japanese people may transform a desirable goal pursued by value rationality into a viable option. To put it another way, this may be regarded as a type of adaptation to values under specific institutional constraints (Merton 1968). More specifically, where conformity to social norms is strict and sanctions against deviation are severe, an actor will take actions that are not necessarily faithful to his or her values and beliefs. All in all, the influence of value-rationality on a choice of action is affected by institutional settings in society.

The second implication is that human attitudes change in a flexible way. As the results of the analysis in Chap. 5 show, for instance, women's attitudes to inter-generational relations became increasingly individualistic up to birth cohorts born in the early 1960s, after which their attitudes took a sharp turn and shifted towards less individualistic opinions again. It thus follows that attitudes between generations do not always change in a unilineal way. As mentioned in Chap. 2, the theories of a value shift, more or less, tend to hold that inter-generational changes in the beliefs, values, and motivations of people proceed in a single direction (Inglehart 1977, 1990; Inglehart and Baker 2000; Inglehart and Welzel 2005). More specifically, it is implicitly assumed that unprecedented material affluence brought by economic development causes irreversible change in values and beliefs. This may be the case with the ideational theory (Lesthaeghe 1983; Lesthaeghe and Meekers 1986; Lesthaeghe and Surkyn 1988; Lesthaeghe and Vanderhoeft 2001; van de Kaa 1994, 2001). More specifically, the theory tends to postulate that the decline of traditional values and the emphasis on individualism occur across developed countries. Yet, this unilineal model of evolution does not hold true in Japanese society. From a long-term perspective, after the individualistic attitudes within birth cohorts strengthened, they became weak again in Japan. This evidence leads us to think that a value shift is more flexible and reversible than the ideational theory assumes. In other words, we may dare to say that each society has its own path of ideational change.

6.8 Towards a Comparative Institutional Analysis of Marriage and Fertility

Throughout the course of this study, we have attempted to examine marriage and fertility behaviour in Japan. The results of this study challenge some aspects of the economic and the ideational theories. For instance, while economic status affects marriage patterns, the influence of values and beliefs is not so strong in Japan as to cause a similar change in marriage behaviour in North-Western Europe. This leads us to further consideration of the relation between demographic behaviour and institutions. Admittedly, institutions may be described as an endogenous outcome of an economic game (Morgan et al. 2010). At the same time, however, institutions can be regarded as a set of constraints that actors generally follow (North 1990, 2005). Adopting the latter definition of institutions, we can argue that institutional settings circumscribe a range of behavioural choices in a society (see Chap. 2). For instance, let us imagine a society that demands strong conformity to conventional values and lifestyles, and imposes material and psychological sanctions against deviation from established norms. In such a society, even if people have more progressive and self-centred attitudes in mind, most of them will not dare to disobey conventional forms of behaviour. In this case, ideational factors will have a relatively weak impact on marriage and fertility behaviour. In other words, theoretical frameworks of instrumental- and value-rationality are useful in depicting the motivational side of demographic behaviour. The actual impact of economic and ideational factors on marriage and fertility patterns is, however, affected by an institutional environment within a society. Differing institutional settings may serve to bring about wide variation in the effects that economic and attitudinal factors can have on demographic behaviour. Of course, we do not deny that, while institutions constrain actor's conducts, the latter produce and reproduce the former (Aoki 2001, 2007). Taking this point into consideration, we can conclude that more comparative empirical research on marriage and fertility behaviour in various institutional settings is necessary for a further understanding of partnership and family formation in developed countries.

References

Aoki, M. (2001). *Toward a comparative institutional analysis*. Cambridge, Massachusetts: MIT Press.

Aoki, M. (2007). Endogenizing institutions and institutional changes. *Journal of Institutional Economics, 3*, 1–31.

Ariès, P. (1980). Two successive motivations for the declining birth rate in the west. *Population and Development Review, 6*, 645–650.

Goffman, E. (1986). *Frame analysis: An essay on the organization of experience*. Boston: Northeastern University Press.

Inglehart, R. (1977). *The silent revolution: Changing values and political styles among western publics*. Princeton: Princeton University Press.

Inglehart, R. (1990). *Culture shift in advanced industrial society*. Princeton: Princeton University Press.

Inglehart, R., & Baker, W. E. (2000). Modernization, cultural change, and the persistence of traditional values. *American Sociological Review, 65*, 19–51.

Inglehart, R., & Welzel, C. (2005). *Modernizations, cultural change, and democracy: The human development sequence*. Cambridge: Cambridge University Press.

Lesthaeghe, R. (1983). A century of demographic and cultural change in Western Europe. *Population and Development Review, 9*, 411–436.

Lesthaeghe, R., & Camille, V. (2001). Ready, willing, and able: A conceptualization of transitions to new behavioral forms. In John B. C (Ed.), *Diffusion processes and fertility transition* (pp. 240–264).Washington, D.C.: National Academy Press.

Lesthaeghe, R., & Meekers, D. (1986). Value changes and the dimension of familism in the European community. *European Journal of Population, 2*, 225–268.

Lesthaeghe, R., & Surkyn, J. (1988). Cultural dynamics and economic theories of fertility change. *Population and Development Review, 14*, 1–45.

Merton, R. K. (1968). *Social theory and social structure*. New York: Free Press.

Morgan, G., Campbell, J. L., Crouch, C., Pedersen, O. K., & Whitley, R. (Eds.). (2010). *The Oxford handbook of comparative institutional analysis*. Oxford: Oxford University Press.

North, D. C. (1990). *Institutions, institutional change and economic performance*. Cambridge: Cambridge University Press.

North, D. C. (2005). *Understanding the process of economic change*. Princeton: Princeton University Press.

van de Kaa, D. J. (1994). The second demographic transition revisited: Theories and expectations. In G. Beets. (Ed.), *Population and family in the low countries 1993: Late fertility and other current issues* (pp. 81–126). Lisse: Swets & Zeitlinger.

van de Kaa, D. J. (2001). Postmodern fertility preferences: From changing value orientation to new behavour. In edited by R. A. Bulatao & J. B. Casterline (Eds.), *Global fertility transition* (pp. 290–331). New York: Population Council.

Weber, M. (1978a). *Economy and society: An outline of interpretive sociology*. Berkeley: University of California Press.

Weber, M. (1978b). The foundations of social theory. In W. G. Runciman (Ed.), *Max Weber selections in translation* (pp. 3–61). Cambridge: Cambridge University Press.

Weber, M. (2002). *Basic concepts in sociology*. New York: Kensington Publishing.

Zuanna, G. D., & Micheli, G. A. (Eds.). (2004). *Strong family and low fertility: A paradox? New perspectives in interpreting contemporary family and reproductive behaviour*. Dordrecht: Kluwer Academic Publisher.

Author Index

N. Fukuda, *Marriage and Fertility Behaviour in Japan*,
DOI 10.1007/978-981-10-0294-6

Subject Index

N. Fukuda, *Marriage and Fertility Behaviour in Japan*,
DOI 10.1007/978-981-10-0294-6

W

Y

CPSIA information can be obtained at www.ICGtesting.com
Printed in the USA
BVOW06*0220090216

436061BV00004B/13/P

9 789811 002922